Judy Taylor is a schoo
Guide Dogs for the Blind
the blind she was award
January 1989.

She lives in Belper, Derb
sons and two dogs.

JUDY TAYLOR

As I See It

GRAFTON BOOKS

A Division of the Collins Publishing Group

LONDON GLASGOW
TORONTO SYDNEY AUCKLAND

Grafton Books
A Division of the Collins Publishing Group
8 Grafton Street, London W1X 3LA

Published in paperback by Grafton Books 1991
9 8 7 6 5 4 3 2 1

First published in Great Britain by
Grafton Books 1989

A CIP catalogue record for this book is available from
the British Library

ISBN 0–586–20636–1

Printed in Great Britain by
Collins, Glasgow

Set in Palatino

Contents

*To my parents
in gratitude for their wisdom,
love and encouragement*

Preface

Suddenly it hit me with a sharp slap. It was as though I had been standing at the edge of the sea, the tiny ripples of water playing around my ankles, while my bare toes sank comfortably into the warm, soft sand. And then, without warning, the great wave crashed beside me, a sudden, terrifying, cold shock which almost took me off my feet, so unprepared was I for the force of its impact.

'The book' had been around for years, it seemed, almost a part of our home's furnishings. Increasingly, at the end of my talks on the work of the Guide Dogs for the Blind Association, someone in the audience would say, 'You ought to write a book.' I have always written things – just trivial bits of this and that, mostly for my own amusement, or stories for the children when they were small. It would be good, I thought, to have written an account of the lives of the four lovely dogs whose faithful service has been instrumental in enabling me to live the 'normal' sort of life after which I have always striven.

And so it was begun, one Sunday afternoon, several years ago. As it developed, 'the book' became an absorbing weekend hobby which might, some day, serve to amuse my family and friends.

Slowly, Sunday by Sunday, the book evolved, until the routine eye operation which so dramatically altered the course of my life put a temporary stop to its progress. So amazing, though, were some of my thoughts, feelings, and experiences at the time, that I began to keep a diary in which I recorded them.

Astonished by many people's fascination with what had happened to me, I showed the original book to a few friends, one of whom gave it to a literary agent to look at.

Soon after that the big wave came and hit me and jolted me out of my private, comfortable little place there on the warm edge of the sea and sand. I had written an autobiography which was going to be published. How arrogant, how presumptuous that suddenly seemed to me. Who on earth was I, a very ordinary housewife and very part-time teacher, to assume that people would want to read about me? I suddenly felt very vulnerable, too, for in the book I had divulged some of my innermost feelings – feelings I had previously endeavoured to keep to myself.

As I have stated elsewhere in my book, I am neither clever nor brave. I have known, and heard of, other people with disabilities who have done far more outstanding things with their lives than I have done. What, then, do I consider to be the purpose, or purposes of this book?

It has been my practice, when speaking on the subject of guide dogs and the wonderful job they do, to try to give my audiences an insight into the lives of people who are disabled in one way or another, and to help them to understand that those who have some sort of disability are simply human beings like themselves, with normal emotions, hopes and aspirations who just want to get on and live their lives as fully as possible. I dare to hope that this book, too, will help readers to feel at ease when they come alongside people who have disabilities. I hope the book shows that a disability does not need to be looked upon as an all-engulfing tragedy, but that some of the old prejudices can have a disabling effect upon those who are striving to live a normal life.

I think that, since human nature is complex, and most

of us are different people at different times, this is not a book just about me. I think it is about many of you who will read it. I hope you will all find some comfort or encouragement in its pages.

Last of all, this book is a 'thank you': to the Guide Dogs for the Blind Association for Neana, Dana, Martin and Victor; the Royal National Institute for the Blind; the Amber Valley Social Services; the Derbyshire Association for the Blind; the Amber Valley Talking Newspapers for the Blind; and Mr H. Salem and all staff at the Derbyshire Royal Infirmary. Many others are mentioned with special gratitude during the unfolding of the narrative. On the other hand, some dearly loved friends do not appear. This does not indicate a lack of regard for them, or of appreciation of the part they have played in my life. It is simply a result of narrative compression.

I must also mention the countless numbers, whose names I shall never know, who gave a few moments to assist at busy road crossings, helped out on train journeys or in restaurants and other public places. These are 'the ships that pass in the night' who would probably never guess how much their brief offer of companionship has helped to ease my way through life's journey.

CHAPTER 1

Home and School

Although I was unable to appreciate it at the time, I realize in retrospect that my very humble beginnings laid far stronger foundations for my life than a more sheltered environment could ever have done.

My parents, Phyllis and Frederick Harris, both bright and both members of very large families, had passed scholarship exams in their childhood, but in those days working-class children from large families could rarely afford to take up the offer of a grammar-school education. My mother and father had both started work at the age of fourteen, and the Depression of the thirties had made its mark upon them. They have always claimed that their luck turned at my birth in 1935, as from that time Dad was never again to be out of work, although his weekly earnings kept us only just above the poverty line.

It was regarded, however, as a definite step up in life when we moved from the cottage in the hamlet of Hempsted, near Gloucester, with no electricity or sanitation, and the risk of the Severn using it as part of its bed each spring, to a small terraced house in a cul-de-sac in the less salubrious quarter of Cheltenham.

My bright blue-grey eyes betrayed nothing of the fact which was later to prove the greatest single determining factor of the way in which my life would go. But as I grew from baby to toddler, and on into childhood, it became plain that all was not well, and by the time I was four it had been established that a then unidentified eye condition would eventually lead to my becoming totally blind. There is no history of blindness in our family, and we can only assume that the very severe attack of measles I had at the age of thirteen months damaged various parts of my eyes. It was not until I was able to walk that my parents ever suspected that anything was wrong. Mum tells me that, at first, she used to get quite impatient with me when I bumped into things, until it became obvious that I simply hadn't seen them.

My sight deteriorated so gradually that, until I was nine, I attended the local school and managed to take an active part in most of what went on there. How grateful I am that during those formative years I had a strong awareness of the beauties of nature. During my many years of blindness I retained a vivid memory of the deep blue of a summer sky, with fluffy white clouds like great wisps of thistledown, and the rich lush green of trees in full leaf. And when on autumn days I walked ankle-deep in fallen leaves, I immediately saw in my mind's eye those rich autumnal hues of rust and orange and deep coppery yellow. My dreams at night were often full of visual detail, which I could recall easily. I treasured these early visual memories, for they brought the world of what is seen very close to me.

That shabby little back street, with its rough, unmade road and almost non-existent pavements, with its tiny houses, whose doors opened straight upon the street, where there were no cars, because no one who lived there could have afforded such a luxury; this street, with its few hens scratching about on a piece of waste land in the corner, might seem to an outsider to have had little to recommend itself as a place where one might choose to live. But to the young, inquisitive minds of us children, it had a wondrous magical quality all of its own. What really lay behind those huge double doors that almost spanned the entire width of the street beyond number nine? We only managed to snatch a brief glimpse into the mysterious shadowiness as the greengrocer, whose shop was on the main road, opened them to drive his van through each evening. None of us was awake when he drove out in the morning. What could be the cause of the occasional bursts of laughter from the groups of men who smoked and sometimes spat – how grown-up and daring that seemed – on the corners outside the pubs? And what forbidden, mysterious things did the grannies and younger women discuss, their heads together, nodding knowingly as they knitted on, giving each other looks full of meaning, and placing warning fingers upon tight-buttoned lips if our ball should roll too near the huddled group? This was a wonderful place in which to live, full of vibrant, real, heart-beat life. It would be hard to imagine anywhere on earth which could have stimulated and challenged the body and mind of a lively little handicapped child more than here. Here I was unconditionally accepted.

Perhaps in 'Please Mr Wolf, may I cross the river?' I was caught and 'on' rather more often than the others; and certainly it was wise to keep your distance if I happened to be joining in games on bikes. I did actually achieve one title in our street – I was the champion lamp-post climber. I could get to the very top of the lamp-post outside our front door. It wasn't until many years later that I realized I had an unfair advantage: if I looked down, I couldn't see how far away the pavement was.

But for me it wasn't like that all the time – only in our street. Sometimes life was hellish.

After one of the interminable monthly visits to the eye clinic, where we seemed to spend hours shuffling along the shiny benches on our bottoms, I was informed that I would have to wear glasses. How I dreaded the arrival of the parcel containing the ugly little round spectacles with their thin silvery frames. And from the moment I made my first appearance in them at school, the teasing and taunting began. 'Four eyes, four eyes', some of the rough boys chanted, and 'Blind as a bat', they would hiss, out of earshot of the teachers. I could only stand there, the nasty little culprits pinching my nose and hurting my ears, the two thick discs of glass improving my sight not at all and in no way hiding the tears of shame that welled up behind them. 'Specky Four-eyes, blind as a bat', they chorused, enjoying themselves enormously as they danced around me, twitching the point of my pixie-hood until they had tugged it from my head. I could do little to prevent these tauntings. Every bit of my mind was occupied with concentrating on the dimly seen pavement, watching out for holes in the road, and half-looking, half-listening for oncoming cars. Beyond the end of the street I was frightened and alone, because out there I was not accepted, and it was inexplicably lonely being the only one who knew about the bleak helplessness of my situation and the humiliation of being different.

After tea, however, back out in our street, dressed up in our mothers' old clothes, clomping around in their old high-heeled shoes and feeling very grown-up, we rehearsed little shows with which to entertain the long-suffering grannies and the younger women who might have time to watch. We found a book – belonging to someone's elder sister – which made it quite clear that the new babies that arrived in our street from time to time had nothing at all to do with gooseberry bushes or a stork, and we played Hide and Seek around the air-raid shelters. Then the chanting, teasing, bullying boys were quite forgotten, and the little freak with the nasty silvery spectacles was just an ordinary little girl again – accepted, included, and safe.

In the little spare room at the end of our landing I could

be truly safe and secure. Being different didn't matter there, because in there I could be anything I wished to be. It didn't matter that the plaster on the walls was crumbling – that was only the way that grown-ups saw it. Your eyes had to be good, like everyone else's, normal eyes, to see such ordinary things. When your eyes were 'different', you could make that room into anything you liked. It was a secret, romantic place, at the top of a fairy castle. Because I couldn't see the shabby little backyards through the window, there was no problem about imagining them as exotic gardens full of bright flowers and butterflies. Even the fun of street games paled into insignificance as, having wound up the old gramophone and placed the needle upon the first groove, I heard the scratchy, boxed-up voice from somewhere deep inside sing out into the friendly air of this safe little kingdom, 'Smoke Gets in Your Eyes' and 'Dancing Cheek to Cheek'. They were grown-ups' songs, and I didn't understand, most of the time, what they were all about, but it didn't matter. The tunes were full of enchantment and make-believe and, dressed in something borrowed from Mum's wardrobe – probably her wedding veil with its waxy orange-blossom – I could dance and whirl around as the notes from the gramophone rose and fell in tinny cascades of melody. I could whirl and twirl as fast as I cared to, for if I tripped or bumped into things there, there was no one to scoff and jeer.

In the little spare room I could have real dignity, for there was no one to take it away. Only Willy went in there with me. Willy was a ginger cat with a funny, bent tail. They said that someone had trapped it in a door; and they also said he had been taken away from his mother too soon. The backyard cats didn't like him, because he was different, too, but I loved him more than almost anything in the world. When the boys at school had been particularly unkind, I would bury my face in his soft, warm fur, and tell him all about it. His little, pointed ears would twitch, he would flick his funny bent tail and purr louder than I have ever heard any other cat purr. I knew that he understood all those things that ached right down inside me, for in his animal way, he had suffered them too.

We kept these things as secrets between ourselves, my feline friend and I. Then, suddenly becoming aware that the grating, scratchy, tinny, wondrous strains of 'Smoke Gets in Your Eyes' were getting slower and slower, and descending alarmingly through key after key, the necessity to jump up and wind up the gramophone again before it ground to a crunching halt jolted us straight back into the world of reality and 'normal' ordinariness, and 'Time for tea'.

English summers are lovely, but short, and the summer of my early childhood was short, too. I did not, however, have the luxurious time of rich autumn with its gradually declining sun and the soft humming of tired bees and scents of ripening fruits and browning leaves to lead me gently from laughing summer into winter's chill. When I was nine the dark clouds dropped suddenly, and the air chilled all at once, like a great icy hand plucking my small life out of its secure homeliness, snatching away all that was dear and loved and familiar. 'She will have to go away to a special school for blind children,' the social worker told my mother in a matter-of-fact way. By this time I was certainly struggling at school, for I could no longer see the print in books, and could read work on the blackboard only with the greatest difficulty.

On a morning in January, Mum and I walked out of our little street to board the train and steam off into a new, unknown life. Never again would I really be a part of the street, the games, the long summer evenings. I would from now on always be on the outside, for they had 'sent me away to school'.

The place was austere, although very clean and efficiently run. We were certainly not treated unkindly, and were adequately, if not imaginatively, fed. Everything, though, appeared to me to be regimented, and every situation seemed to be accompanied by a list of rules. The dormitory in which I slept held beds for thirty children, fifteen along each side, and a stool between each bed.

Within minutes of arrival, all my own clothes were taken away, rolled into a neat bundle, clearly labelled and stowed away in the 'wardrobe room'. Pretty dresses and soft woolly jumpers were exchanged for a set of grey garments. In summer, the only difference was that itchy grey blouses had short instead of long sleeves, and itchy grey ankle socks replaced winter's grey knee-socks. We moved in a silent, orderly file as shrill blasts of a whistle summoned us in turn to meals, lessons, chapel and bed.

Visiting days were few and far between. I hardly dared look forward to seeing my mother, knowing, before she arrived, the agony that would have to be borne when the few precious hours had passed and she must go away again, leaving me a part of the greyness, the silent lines and the oh, so clean, but completely unfriendly, hard little bed in its neat row.

Nevertheless, I realized even then that the teachers were dedicated to their work, and I do owe the school two eternal debts of gratitude. Firstly, I learned to read Braille. Even as a very small child I had always been an avid reader and had been frustrated, as my sight deteriorated, to have to wait for others to read to me; people rarely seemed able to spare the time, or not enough to satisfy my voracious appetite for stories. How eagerly I applied myself to the task of learning to interpret the symbols formed by the little dots. How thrilling it was, as my fingers became more and more sensitive, to find the dots beginning to spring out as words, and those words become the fabric of stories. There was also a girl in my dormitory who had a fair degree of sight, and on summer evenings, when we knew the staff were at supper, she would read to us from books hidden under her mattress. The adventures of Enid Blyton's 'Famous Five' filled my mind so completely that for at least half an hour even the unfriendly smell of the stiff, laundered sheets was forgotten.

And, secondly, there was music.

It was at this school that I had my first piano and violin lessons, and after a little while was allowed to sing in the choir in chapel. I sat in the back row of trebles, and trembled with excitement as the organ boomed out the introduction of some great chorus by Handel, Bach or Stainer and we stood waiting to take that deep breath and then the great, lovely harmonies soared higher and higher weaving webs of sound that made me feel that, even there, heaven could not be too far away. And then there were the half-hours in the practising rooms, when I was blessedly alone, not part of the ever-present crowd, but not lonely, as I was at night, horribly lonely in that small hard bed in its neat row.

CHAPTER 2

Chorleywood

When I was almost eleven, the headmaster sent for my parents and suggested that I should take an examination which, if I passed, would enable me to continue my education at Chorleywood College, a grammar school for blind and partially-sighted girls.

Having passed the examination in the summer of 1946, I set out on this new adventure in the September after my eleventh birthday, and spent what were probably seven of the happiest years of my life in that lovely old house, built in the style of a French château, and sensitively converted for use as a school. Panelled rooms with great open fireplaces in which logs burned on winter evenings, a great sweeping oak staircase, a winter garden with a wrought-iron staircase and balcony and still a few exotic plants, french windows opening on to lawns which swept down to tennis courts, and mysterious shrubberies with great old cedar trees, all gave me a feeling of belonging to a bygone age of gracious living and almost of being a part of some romantic tale from the past. In the dormitories, each with no more than half-a-dozen beds, there were dressing-tables, pretty bedside rugs and counterpanes, and even wardrobes where we kept our own clothes for wearing on Wednesday, Saturday and Sunday afternoons.

This unique school had been the brainchild of Miss Phyllis Monk, who felt that blind and partially-sighted girls should have an opportunity to enter the professions, and that an education which would equip them for such careers should be available. Leaving a secure teaching post in a public school for girls, she launched into this venture with much faith but little financial security, and a handful of young charges. In a comparatively short time she was able to house her growing number of pupils in The Cedars, as it was originally called, and the school remained there until the late 1980s, a memorial to her courage and faith. I had the honour of meeting Miss Monk once, long after she had retired, when several of us in the sixth form were invited for tea in her cottage nearby. I believe she was a Quaker, and peace and serenity flowed from her like liquid light. I am sure she must have had a very beautiful face. She was, I think, the most gracious person I have ever met, and although she had retired some years before I arrived at the school, something of her aura was still there in all the rooms and along the shrubbery walks.

My memories of those first months at Chorleywood are hazy. I remember being astonished that a school could smell of wax polish, scented soap and baking. The school cat, with her little hunched back, thought her own thoughts, but stopped occasionally on her prowls around the great house, and waited long enough to be stroked, reminding me of cosiness and home; but here I thought of home with affection rather than grief.

The school's philosophy was years ahead of its time. Application to classroom studies and academic achievement were, of course, enormously important. But it was considered equally, if not more, important that each girl should achieve a rounded personality and have a healthy attitude towards her handicap and her future life in the world so that she could fit in unobtrusively and serve the community usefully. Great stress was put upon developing an independent attitude, and a spirit of adventure was encouraged. These were excellent lessons for life, and have served me well through the ups and downs of everyday living.

The beautiful house in its extensive park-like grounds stood in lovely rolling countryside, on the edge of a bracken-covered common. A short path across the common led to the parish church, which we all attended on Sunday mornings, and a longer path through the bracken and across more open country led to the village about a mile away. Here there were several shops where we were able to spend our pocket money. For the first two years we went out every day, accompanied by a teacher; there would be a dozen of us together, walking two by two. We thoroughly explored our surroundings – common, village, fields, lanes and woods – until every square foot for miles around was so familiar that I believe I would have noticed if one bush had been uprooted, or one sapling had disappeared.

During one of these excursions my partner, who had some sight, stopped to look in a shop-window in the village. Suddenly we realized that we were alone, and quickened our pace, hoping to catch the others up unnoticed. Alas, crossroads ahead made it quite impossible to be certain of ever finding the 'croc' before our absence had been discovered. A man coming towards us gave us a cheery 'Good afternoon.' Imagine his thoughts when we responded with the question, 'Have you seen a crocodile walking along this way?' 'I'm afraid not,' he replied, quickening his pace and, I suspect, getting away as fast as he could.

After this period of initiation, so long as written permission from parents was obtained, we could spend these hours in the open air with a partner of our choice. Later we would be allowed to go by bus to the nearby town of Rickmansworth on Saturday afternoons to shop and we were also allowed to choose our place of worship on Sundays.

This choice, I must admit, perhaps with a little shame, was not always guided by the most spiritual of reasons. In the village there was a small chapel with an incredibly wheezy organ and an even wheezier 'sing leader'. The musical interludes made this place of worship well worth a visit. I'm afraid we hardly even tried to suppress our mirth as organ and soprano rose together in an agonized top G. The congregation was made up of warm, loving people, who were very kind to us, and Christianly overlooked our misdemeanours.

In spite of this shocking lack of reverence during organized worship I was a deeply religious child, and loved to retreat to the peace of the little chapel the staff and girls had made together in an alcove of the old wine cellars beneath the house. In its solitude I could find myself, the real 'me', who lived somewhere deep inside, refusing most of the time to appear in public, hiding behind the façade of practical jokes and often opinionated views on all manner of subjects. I believe that at this time I was not an easy sort of child. The real 'me' within had been badly bruised. An independent spirit had been locked away just long enough for scars to show and, like a butterfly, the 'me' with whom I had almost lost touch would settle until the hand tried to close, and then flit away and hide. But in the quietness beneath the house, where there were always fresh flowers on the little altar, I knew that God knew where I was, and I was able to rest in that knowledge, without completely understanding it.

We were great practical jokers, the little group of which I was a part. I suppose the pranks we played would seem tame to the more sophisticated youth of today, but it was always clean fun, never hurtful or cruel.

I remember sneaking one evening into the staff cloakroom to procure the coat of the tallest teacher – she was over six feet tall and until you got to know her seemed a formidable character. We 'borrowed' a long stilt from the games cupboard, made a somewhat grotesque cardboard face, attached this and a coathanger to the stilt in the appropriate places, and decked it out with the coat. Just for good measure, we fixed a Latin textbook under the coatsleeve so that no one should be confused as to the identity of the figure.

On another occasion we made an effigy of Matron, using pillows, rolled-up Braille *Radio Times* for the limbs, and 'borrowed' or contrived articles of her uniform. This we sat as upright as the floppy pillow would allow on the loo in her bathroom and somehow rigged a string from the doorhandle to the lavatory chain so that, when she entered this private chamber, the action of closing the door behind her caused the chain to be pulled. We never did hear of her reaction. The incident was not mentioned.

And then, of course, there were from time to time those midnight feasts which did dreadful things to the adrenalin. Food would be procured from the village and hidden in cake tins. A dressing-table in our dormitory had been conveniently placed across the opening of a large fireplace, and this made an excellent hidy-hole for all sorts of things. At half-past ten, when the corridor lights were turned off, we covered the floor with our counterpanes to muffle any sounds of movement and retrieved the goodies from the fireplace. If it had just been a civilized hand-out of food to be eaten before we retired to our beds, all would have been well; but some of our number became over-daring, spirits grew high, chatter and laughter broke out and almost always we were caught, the remains of the feast were confiscated, and we had to face, the next day, the ignominy of standing before everyone in assembly and outlining to them the nature of our offence. Our innocent adventure

acquired a different complexion when such words as
deceitful, dishonest, and irresponsible were linked with
it. But however dampened at the time, we lived to hold
many more such revelries and fearfully enjoyed every
one of them.

Hard play was balanced by hard study. Most of the
subjects taught at an ordinary grammar school were
offered here, and taken by all to O-level standard and
right through to A-level by many of the girls. We
followed the normal course in languages, history and
scripture; in maths, science and geography we used
equipment specifically designed for the blind, such as
raised maps, and bells instead of lights to indicate that
certain experiments had been successfully accomplished.

There was much music-making, we had our own
Guide and Ranger groups, and a very active drama group
which in summer staged many very creditable open-air
productions by anyone's standards, in a lovely natural
stage setting among the trees by the shrubbery. At one
time there were hens, ducks, a pony, a donkey and a
lamb to be cared for on a rota system, watched over by
the gym teacher. I was more than a little apprehensive of
her at the time, but in later years, I realized we all owed
her much. She persuaded, coaxed, and sometimes even
shamed us a little into doing all sorts of things that at that
time most people would not have thought possible in a
school for visually handicapped children.

Twice a term we had 'At Home' evenings, in which we
were all expected to take part. Some would play
instruments, some sing, and others recite poems or act
short plays. After an invitation out to tea by a family in
the neighbourhood, and this was not uncommon, we
were taught to write a 'thank you' letter before a day had
passed. 'Your left hand is for bread and butter, and your

right for your teacup', we were instructed, if the offending right hand inadvertently strayed towards the bread plate.

As London was less than twenty miles away, we were encouraged to enjoy all that the capital had to offer in the way of culture and entertainment. There were visits to the Science Museum, concerts at the Royal Albert Hall and the Festival Hall, and Shakespeare plays at the Old Vic and in the open air at Regent's Park. What a busy life, but very good, oh, very good indeed.

My form was small by ordinary standards: there were about ten of us, but that was not an uncommon number in special schools. Indeed, when we were all taking notes, or writing essays, on our Braille writing machines, I doubt whether the normal human ear could reasonably have been expected to cope with a greater number of decibels. Our academic abilities ranged from very nearly brilliant to fairly mediocre. I do not believe that I fitted into either category, most certainly not the former. The great Creator had, however, endowed me with perhaps more than my fair share of creative gifts, and I use the word advisedly. I have come to look upon every good thing we have as a gift, and while I am more than willing to respect the views of others, which may differ from mine, I do not believe in 'rights'.

By the time I was twelve, I had discovered an unusual facility for turning a lump of clay into animal and human forms which were very realistic. The same applied to pieces of material and paper, which were rapidly and accurately transformed into a great variety of objects, both useful and decorative. I loved to feel the different media changing in my fingers and becoming something that had started somewhere deep down inside my thoughts and feelings.

Another of my passions at that time was to become, if

only temporarily, completely and entirely another being from myself, and this I did through drama. Many of our staff were very creative in this sphere and we staged dramatic productions several times a year. I was rarely happier than when made up and dressed as a character for such a performance: I stepped right outside myself, looked out at the world through the eyes of another, and breathed life into one who may have lived long ago or, indeed, may never have lived at all.

I am not exactly sure when Lyndall Frost joined the staff at Chorleywood. A quietly colourful character, who made a deep impression upon me, she came principally to teach drama, but was gifted in many other spheres. The talented staff had brought out in us an ability to cope with a full-blown production of a play by, say, Shakespeare or Shaw, the standard of which surprised many an audience: Miss Frost added a new dimension of professionalism to this well-turned earth. Some of us were entered for public examinations in poetry-speaking and drama. As I threw myself into the character of Saint Joan for one of these exams and Catherine Howard, in *A Rose Between Two Thorns*, for a school entertainment, I felt that acting was what I wanted to do more than anything else in the world.

I spoke to Miss Frost about it. We discussed the matter at length. In those days there was not much talk about equality for disabled people. It was pointed out that, even if I were accepted by a college and trained in the dramatic arts, I would most probably have only curiosity value as a professional actress, and few prospects of a lasting career. I think that was good advice. At college I took drama as one of my main subjects and had a part in two plays. After that I locked that ambition away with other memories too precious to risk having them damaged by people's incredulity or disbelief.

And then there was that other great and lasting love – music. I continued to play the piano and violin, and added the organ to these for a short time, but took little pleasure in that. As we were so near London, we attended many first-rate concerts. Everything about these occasions was thrilling to me. I breathed in the smell of a concert hall, a smell I cannot describe, but which has not changed at all as the years have gone by. Like the legendary Chinese visitors who are supposed to have applauded after the orchestra finished tuning up, I was thrilled to the core as the instruments sharpened and flattened offending notes, and ran up and down rapid scales. And then there was that vibrant hush before the conductor began to unfold wave after wave of sound, rising and falling, clutching at the heartstrings, awakening in the soul joys and sorrows almost too beautiful to be contained.

Yet what use were these gifts for a future career? I think most of the staff assumed that I would become a musician, but I knew even then that I lacked that extra something which would have been necessary for a career in music. Anyway, life was far too full of fun to spend time agonizing over what, after all, was nothing more than a rather irritating necessity in the future: who wants to be concerned about the future when the present is so good?

I never considered going to university, and I am not sure whether this was because I did not rate my academic abilities highly enough or simply that I did not fancy the industry and application involved. Looking back, I have always slightly regretted this.

I feel certain that the years of adolescence were made neither more nor less difficult by my disability. Few teenagers sail quite unaffected through those years when they are too old to be classed as children and yet too young for their opinions to be taken quite seriously by the adult world. I feel that I can say, quite truthfully, that even then I had few hang-ups about my blindness. On the whole, I was satisfied with my lot and felt that even had I had full sight my way of life would have been little changed. True, I would not have had to go to boarding school, but I loved my school, and have never regretted at all the years I spent there.

I think that I probably looked forward with equal excitement to the moment when, stepping from the train, I would be met either by Mum at the beginning of the school holidays or at Paddington by a teacher who, having met girls from several trains about the same time, would conduct her charges, chattering excitedly, safely back to start the new term.

When we got home, Mum and I always chuckled because, on the walk from the station, we invariably met someone we knew who, on seeing me, would ask Mum, 'How is she? And when is she going back?' My mother was almost as sensitive as I was about this business of talking to me through a third person, and usually said that since she had only just met me, she didn't really have too much information about the state of my well-being, and suggested that they asked me in person.

It was lovely to be at home with my parents and little brother. Nicholas was born at Christmas, eleven months after I first went away to school, and I was allowed to choose his second name, Jeffrey. That was a strange Christmas: Dad was abroad, serving with the RAF, and the new little bundle in the cot in the corner seemed to need a great deal of attention. The shock of my comparative unimportance just then was only softened by Mum's Christmas present to me – my first violin. I feel sure, in retrospect, that matters were no easier for Nick as the years went by and I came home for school holidays, assuming the role of head sibling and bossing him shamefully. In spite of this, an unwritten code of love grew between us and we knew we could trust each other with our deepest secrets.

However happy I was to be with my family, at times I was very lonely. The friends of my childhood had drifted away, and I soon began to long for the kind of fun and laughter that we share only with our peers.

Our house, at that time, was next to a huge playing field. Some time during August, a huge fair came there for a week. I could just make out from my bedroom window the lights of the big wheel, high up in the air, and I could hear the music, all the latest tunes, playing on and on until long after dark. Occasional peals of laughter conjured up in the mind's eye a picture of boys and girls with bright, laughing faces, running here and there in the bustling, hot, noisy atmosphere. I would stand at my bedroom window, my heart aching. How I longed to be ordinary, and one of them. If they knew about me, I wondered, would they come for me, and let me be one of the noisy, laughing crowd?

Things were immensely improved, though, after I joined the Air Rangers. Once they realized that, in spite of my handicap, I was perfectly human and experienced the same joys and sorrows as they, I made friends with a couple of the girls and did not feel so cut off from my contemporaries during the school holidays.

During the holidays just before O-levels I announced to my somewhat surprised parents that I was going to become a telephonist. My father, rather inconveniently for me, asked me to explain this decision. Now, while I would never describe myself as a very virtuous individual, I must say that I have always been extremely honest – perhaps too honest sometimes for the comfort of others and my own personal advancement in life. This was one such occasion. Quite truthfully, I confessed that my only reason for choosing that particular job lay in the fact that someone had told me that I could be trained to do it in three months, and I knew of no other career with such a short period of initiation.

My father, who had been brought up somewhat according to the standards of the Victorian era, looked at me sternly (and his looks could be felt even when not actually seen) and said in a tone which allowed no argument: 'You get back to school and go on studying until you find a better reason than that for deciding about the future. Your mother and I haven't made all these sacrifices for you to decide on the first thing that comes into your head.'

When Dad spoke like that, I didn't even *have* second thoughts, let alone voice them. The sacrificial bit puzzled me rather, but I didn't think it expedient to delve into that too deeply. So back to school I went, took and passed a respectable number of O-levels, and returned the following year to enter the sixth form.

CHAPTER 3

College

In the summer of the following year, 1952, I had the experience which was to change my whole life and set its course for many years to come.

It was hot and sunny, one of those perfect June days when, feeling the dappled sunlight through the leaves on the trees, and listening to the lazy droning of insects, I could dream that everything would be warm and friendly for ever. I was sitting in an alcove at the edge of the lawn which swept down to the ha-ha with its rustic bridge and the tennis courts beyond. The book on my knee did little to excite my attention – I was revising for a geography exam.

Suddenly I was surrounded by a power which gripped my whole attention and took over all of my being. I heard no voice booming from the clouds, but what I knew right then was far stronger and more powerful than any mere feeling. I knew without any doubt that I was to become a teacher, and that I was to teach sighted, not blind, children.

For some time I was quite unable to move. Never at any time of my life had I contemplated teaching as a career. It must be something to do with the sun, and perhaps after tea, when the air was cooler, I would feel better. But no, this new knowledge would not go away. I hardly slept that night, and the sense of reality that morning brings after a storm-tossed night did nothing to alter things. A choice had been made on my behalf and, unlikely as it seemed, I knew it had to be.

I related the experience to the head of the school. Miss

McHugh epitomized for me calmness and wisdom. She never wasted words, but seemed to weigh them carefully and they always came out in correct measure. She was a devout Christian, who lived her beliefs, who never preached, but taught so much of what she believed. After listening to my tale, she stated quite calmly that she believed that God had chosen to reveal His will for my life in this way, and although she knew of no other totally blind person who had entered the teaching profession through an ordinary teacher training college, we were to spare no effort in making this course possible for me.

Letters were written to training colleges in many parts of the country, and soon we received a reply from the Principal of St Gabriel's, a college in south-east London, offering me an interview. My memories of that interview are hazy. I know that I wore a brown outfit, including a hat, which I thought added a tone of respectability and sobriety to the general impression. I only remember one question they asked me: 'Why do you want to be a teacher?' 'Oh, I don't *want* to be a teacher,' I replied, the old honesty popping up as usual without thinking, 'I've just *got* to be one.' They couldn't have been too shocked – I was offered a place for the following September.

Now began a completely new chapter in my life. During the next two years I trained to become a teacher, but I believe that during that time I received a more intensive period of training for life itself than ever before or since. It was then that I came slowly to realize the degree to which my personality was affected by my blindness, and in turn how much the acceptance of the handicap depended upon the degree to which I allowed my personality to have its own way. The two were inextricably bound up and neither could be truly dealt with until this fundamental fact had been admitted and accepted by me. I was slow and reluctant to accept; although we had been encouraged at Chorleywood to develop a healthy attitude towards our circumstances, it was not until I was eighteen that I was to feel the full shock of the outside world's attitudes and reactions. As a child in the street at home, I had been fully accepted with the lack of sophistication which characterizes young children; at school I had been protected by being one of many; now I was on my first day at teacher training college, one of 200 young women, and the only one who was blind.

I believe the shock was as great to the other 199 students as it was to me. Most of them had never met a blind person before, let alone one of their own age who wanted only to merge with the crowd. My hearing and other senses, which had long been accustomed to obtaining information about the environment in which I found myself, did their work, and it was not long before I was thoroughly familiar with my surroundings and knew every inch of this large building. There were tell-tale changes in floor surface, small echoes, variations in the circulation of air, all of which gave me the clues upon which I had so long relied to orientate myself. Finding doorways, staircases and turns in the corridors soon became second nature to me. There is, too, a strange, inexplicable feeling around the lower leg which warns of furniture, such as chairs and low tables.

How helpful all those somewhat shocked young women really meant to be. As I approached doors, stairs, or furniture, there were many hands grabbing at me from all directions, and warnings that at times amounted almost to panic that one more step and I would most certainly plunge to an untimely end. And then, with the apparently very common assumption held by much of the world's population that those who are blind must also have seriously impaired hearing, and are probably, just for good measure, not quite right in the head, there were the very audible concerns on my behalf as to how I was ever to cope with a class, mark books or know what the children in my care were up to. All very understandable, I admit, but at that time I was no wiser than they. After all, my only reason for being there at all was that for once in my life I was being completely obedient. I knew that all would be revealed, but had not the vaguest notion at that time as to the nature of the revelation.

Like the majority of teenagers, one of my greatest needs at this time was to conform. No one had hinted to me that, for a blind girl, conformity in a world of sighted people would be a near impossibility without some very radical changes of attitude. And so I began a great pretence. I actually pretended sometimes that I could see. I picked up my Braille books, and peered at the invisible dots while feeling them slyly with my fingers. Waiting for a friend, I would look this way and that up and down the road and when we visited art galleries I would try to make intelligent remarks about paintings.

The greatest trial of all lay in the fact that the hostel in which I lived was about a mile away from the college, and the route between them ran through fairly busy London streets. There were always plenty of offers to 'take' me to and fro, but to have accepted would have been to admit to non-conformity and defeat. With misguided, stubborn independence, I often refused well-meant offers of help and I did not even consider using a white stick – that would have embarrassed me dreadfully. Somehow I managed to make the journey more or less safely, but oh, the strain upon every nerve within me: no words could convey it.

There were those poor unsuspecting window-cleaners and painters, somewhere up towards the sky, going about their business at some third-storey window, quite understandably believing the bottom had dropped out of their world as the ladder, upon which all their confidence lay, was almost knocked from beneath them. My apologies and protestations did little to make up for the strong chances of a heart attack taking place three storeys above my sore and bruised head. Then there were always old dogs who chose the middle of the pavement for a siesta on warm days. They were singularly unimpressed when, disturbed by my falling headlong over their recumbent bodies, I tried to explain politely that it would never have happened if I had been able to see them. I usually did not wait long enough to hear all they had to say to me.

Worst of all, though, was the London traffic, even on the side roads. I would wait at the edge of the kerb and on they would come, one vehicle after another with never a break, just nose, tail, nose, tail, and the occasional loud horn, just to break the monotony of it all. At length, I would shut my eyes, clench my teeth and fists, breathe a quick prayer, and dash for it. Almost always, two steps into the road, I would be stopped by a car pulling up with screeching brakes, inches from my right side. Down would come the window on the driver's side, out would come the head, and then the stream of cockney abuse. Such words. I had never heard most of them, but at least in later years there was never a word overheard in playgrounds full of teenage boys and girls that could shock me – I had heard them all during my years of training, albeit not as part of the college curriculum.

But this self-imposed agony could not go on. The strain of it was taking its toll on my health and nerves. I would arrive at my room after lectures, with studying to do or essays to write, nervously and physically exhausted, able only to throw myself on the bed and sob until I fell asleep.

It was many years before I came fully to realize that one of the signs that a mature and true adjustment to a handicap has taken place is when an offer of help, which may or may not be needed, can be accepted graciously. When I grew older, I never refused help, mostly because I welcomed it, and even if I didn't, because I had come to realize that many people long to feel needed, and I had no right to deny that urge. Eventually I learned, too, to have a sense of humour towards those who treated me as though I were deaf or daft, as well as blind. 'Does she take sugar?' is no myth. It affects us all differently, evoking various reactions. It can undermine a confidence which may already be shaky, in spite of outward appearances. On the other hand, it is sometimes countered by a defensive aggressiveness, which is why some handicapped people may appear to have chips on their shoulders. As the years passed, I became more and more able to laugh about such attitudes, but I am still sometimes caught off guard and make caustic remarks to the one who has delivered the blow.

One day, part-way through the first year at college, a friend decided to take me in hand. She offered no pity, just spoke a few home truths about the folly of my attitude, which was hurting no one but myself, and suggested that I did something constructive, such as getting a guide dog.

I had never thought about a guide dog before, but soon found my mind full of little else. I wrote to the Guide Dogs for the Blind Association requesting speedy delivery of such an animal, and waited for an irregularly shaped parcel. Instead, I received an application form which wanted to know more about me than I felt I knew myself. This was duly filled in and returned. Again I waited for the postman's knock. The next communication was to inform me that my application had been accepted, my name was on the waiting list, and that there would most probably be a suitable dog for me in two years' time.

Although I was disappointed not to have a dog straight away, the fact that I had taken one positive step seemed to make my whole attitude more positive. I realized that if I wanted to be accepted as one of the crowd I had to meet the crowd perhaps even more than half-way. I began to enjoy college life, and all the fun and excitement of being in London. I loved, too, the dazzling lights of the West End, and the crowds pushing their way towards the tube station after a play or show. We used to pay two shillings for the privilege of standing at the back at Sadler's Wells or Covent Garden for a performance of one of the great operas. This was no hardship for me. As I couldn't see the action on the stage anyway, I took a small cushion, or folded my coat, and sat on the floor just soaking up the great embroideries of sound, oblivious of the discomfort and late-comers tripping over my feet.

Once, returning from a dance in a neighbouring college, we found the front door of the hostel locked and barred against us. Even poor Cinderella had been allowed out until midnight, but our revels had to end one hour before hers. Fortunately, a window in the basement had been left unlatched for us by a compassionate fellow student. How grateful we were, but half frightened to death as we clambered through the small opening, for discovery would mean a fine and embarrassing explanations. Through the window climbed the latecomers in their finery – and I was one of them. This fact alone meant more to me even than did the night's fun and music, the young men with whom I had danced, or not danced, and the suppressed giggles which accompanied the nervous late-night break-in. I had been accepted, and was now one of the crowd.

Some of us, decked out in enormous frilly skirts, Spanish shawls and fashionably large earrings, visited the West End coffee bars, popular meeting-places for students. We listened, deeply impressed, while duffle-coated, bearded young men expounded all manner of subjects about which they probably knew nothing at all, but with such intellectual deliberation and long impressive pauses that we hung on their every word, and needed only to look spellbound to please them, and give the impression that we, too, were intellectuals. The fountains in Trafalgar Square, walks through St James's Park and along the Mall, all had a special significance, and I still feel a thrill of excitement when I think of those places.

Some memories are bittersweet. I shall never forget one young man I met at a college dance. We fell into easy conversation, and soon discovered that our interests were very similar. He was a little older than I, and was studying at a college near mine. Having spent so much time chatting to me, he had little choice but to offer to take me back to my hostel. I held his arm, and followed neatly as I felt him going up and down the kerbs on our homeward journey. The talk of music and the teaching career for which we were both training had been stimulating. I felt that our spirits had been in tune. Almost before he could stop himself, he told me that he was going to a concert at the Festival Hall the following week and asked if I would like to go with him. Of course, I accepted.

I took enormous care over my dress for that occasion, and one of my friends helped with my make-up. I must say that I was quite proud of the smoothness with which I stepped on and off the escalators on the underground. I knew that I had not made myself, or him, conspicuous in any way. In the interval, our conversation was animated.

I enjoyed being with this young man and I felt that he enjoyed being with me.

After the concert, we walked along the embankment. It was a hot, still summer night, and the pungent smell of night-scented stocks filled the air. Still chatting comfortably, we sat on a seat beside the river. Suddenly, he stood up, and in a throaty sort of voice informed me that he didn't want to see me again. He told me that he liked me very much – probably too much – and he couldn't allow a friendship that might lead to more grow between himself and a girl who was blind.

I was deeply mortified. I felt that he was telling me that I was sub-standard. I didn't feel sub-standard. Until then I had felt simply like me enjoying myself, remembering the music we had enjoyed, feeling the soft, warm air on my face, smelling the deep, almost exotic aroma of the flowers. I knew I hadn't let him down, hadn't done anything to make him ashamed of being with me, but here he was, embarrassed, telling me he couldn't pursue a relationship he could obviously have enjoyed because, although he didn't put it into words, my blindness made me unacceptable to him. And I never did get around to telling him that, by choice, I wouldn't have gone to a concert, or walked along the embankment, or sat on a seat by the river discussing music and other things, with a man who I had been told had ginger hair and a ginger beard.

Poor young man. Would he, perhaps, have lost face with his friends, with me in tow? 'I have a new girlfriend. She's not bad looking, and has quite a decent figure. I met her at a dance. She seems to know most of the dances and is quite light on her feet. We get on well, and we even like the same kind of music. We had a great evening together. Oh, incidentally, she's blind.'

Poor young man. What a dilemma! If I myself wanted

most of all to merge into the crowd and would use any
ploy in order to achieve that end, it was unreasonable to
expect him to be prepared to stick out like a sore thumb
with his different kind of girlfriend. I bear him no
grudge. It happened many years ago. Time is a great
healer. And who knows, had our positions been
reversed, what might I have done?

Nevertheless, it was a hard blow to my youthful pride,
and I certainly didn't accept it stoically. I kept the pain to
myself, and cried all my hurt into my pillow. I think,
though, that although such reactions to my blindness
never ceased to cause some hurt, it eventually became
little more than an uncomfortable twinge. Little Specky
Four-eyes had been dragged reluctantly from the back
room with its crumbling plaster, its door shut behind her
for ever. Willy, the ginger cat with the bent tail, had been
dead for years, and the wind-up gramophone had long
gone. The time for make-believe was over. She knew that
if she really wanted to be part of the big world, she would
have to come out and learn to face it – its fun and
laughter, and its hard knocks and sorrows, too.

I soon realized, too, that I had not been misled by the
experience in the garden that hot summer day at school.
The studies fascinated me, and in the classroom, on
teaching practice, I knew that I was exactly where I was
supposed to be. The children accepted me, handicap and
all, just for what I was as a person. They did not concern
themselves with the practicalities of how I would cope,
but just got on and left me to manage in whatever way I
pleased. The schools in which we practised were almost
all in very deprived areas of London, south of the river
for the most part, and in them I became aware of poverty
such as I had never known existed. I remember once
asking a class to bring pillowcases for a play we were

doing. They did not respond to the request, and the class teacher told me that most of them probably didn't even have pillows, and to his certain knowledge a number of them slept on the floor, covered by coats. For all that, they were warm, quick and alive, with plenty of initiative, the like of which I have never since encountered. Many of these children had to live on their wits, and they used their wits in all aspects of their lives. Many of the schools were noisy, with street markets outside the classroom windows, and some had playgrounds on the roofs. We worked hard and played hard, and enjoyed both.

The formal side of college life, too, had its own special place and charm. There was formal dinner, for which we were all expected to wear evening dress, and sang Latin grace. We each had turns of sitting at High Table, and once I sat next to the Principal, Dr McKie, who, I am sure, was not as formidable as she appeared to be. There was chapel every morning, and twice on special days. There was much respect for, and adherence to, tradition.

When I embarked upon my college career, the then Ministry of Education agreed to finance my tuition and hostel accommodation, but would not give me a maintenance grant of any kind. The National Institute for the Blind provided me with a typewriter so that I could produce print copies of essays and examination work, and twenty pounds a year to cover the cost of any materials needed because of my blindness. The Institute also paid for the services of a retired teacher who came to read to me books which were unavailable in Braille, and to help me to mark books when we were on teaching practice. Apart from that, I had to survive on fifteen shillings which my parents sent to me each week. That princely sum, which was quite a sacrifice for them, was used to buy my clothes, soap and toothpaste and pay for all entertainment and any meals out. The postal order must have been elastic, for somehow I managed to make it stretch through each week.

At the end of my first year, it came as a great shock to all of us, college staff, my parents, friends, and not least myself, when the Principal received a letter from the Ministry of Education informing her that it was considered an unwise use of the country's money to finance the training for one more year of a blind student who would never be able to qualify.

The Education Officer for Gloucestershire, who gave us a great deal of invaluable support, outlined the position in a letter to my father. It seems that, until then, blind teachers had only worked in schools for the blind, and they had qualified by gaining a university degree. At that time a degree in itself qualified a person to teach. No blind person had been awarded a teaching certificate, the other means of qualifying, and as he said: 'It does not appear to be accepted by the Institute of Education or by the Ministry of Education that a certificate can be granted to a blind student.'

I was not left to face this nightmare alone. Miss McHugh at Chorleywood, the college Principal, Dr McKie, and the heads of the schools in which I had done my teaching practice all wrote very forceful letters on my behalf. They all expressed their conviction of my ability to be a successful teacher if only I were allowed to complete my training. The faceless monster, as it became in my imagination, refused to relent, and further representations from those who supported my case went on for several months. During that summer vacation, my father and I went on foot, or by bus and train, to one official in the educational system after another, each time approaching one a little higher up the ladder than the last, putting our case with simplicity and sincerity.

I felt that my choice of career was God's will, and so, obediently, I fought on. And suddenly, the difficulties were resolved. The path ahead was smooth for a while. The sun shone once more, and my second year at teacher training college began with the Ministry's financial backing. Many thanks to all those dear friends who did not leave me to stumble on alone.

CHAPTER 4

Rugby

My second year in London was as enjoyable and full of new experiences as the first, still evoking in me many treasured memories.

At this time I became involved in a church in the Camberwell area which drew unusually large numbers to its services. The congregation was largely made up of very ordinary south-east London working people. They were wonderfully warm-hearted, always having get-togethers of one kind or another, and I made many new friends. Students from one of the Cambridge colleges had a mission in the parish. Thus, after final examinations, I was included in a parish holiday, held under canvas in Guernsey. What fun we had there, all mucking in together – the clergy, the congregation, Cockney wags, young women from our college and undergraduates from Cambridge. We laughed and sang and drank and danced and prayed together. The summer was hot, and the air was full of the scent of honeysuckle. It was while I was there that the telegram arrived informing me that I had qualified as a teacher, passing one of the three sections of the examination with distinction. Imagine the celebrating that day – and I was excused cookhouse duties, too.

One dark cloud, however, loomed upon the horizon, although for a short space of time I refused to look at it. I had written innumerable letters of application for teaching posts all over the country, always to receive the same sort of reply: 'I am sorry, we do not have a post suitable for you.' I suppose, in retrospect, one can hardly be surprised that head teachers were not able to imagine how a blind teacher could carry out the tasks and duties which that profession would impose, but I felt that they might at least have had a look at me.

By the middle of the summer vacation, all my friends were fixed up with jobs for September, and I could hardly continue to disregard the black cloud ahead. I became depressed and resentful. Resentment is foreign to my personality. I think I can honestly say that I never really resented my blindness. I was sometimes very irritated by the restrictions it imposed, but there was little point in resenting a situation that could not be changed one iota. But just then I was very resentful indeed.

My parents bore the situation stoically, but I knew they were suffering on my behalf. I had wrapped myself in a blanket of gloom which did little to cheer the spirits of those around me. Probably they were somewhat relieved when I told them that I felt a few days in London with a family who had befriended me during my college days would do me good.

How often it has happened in my life that, just as I am sure that the clouds will never again break for me, a shaft of light pierces the darkness. This time the shaft of light came in the form of a completely unexpected letter from Miss Baxter, the headmistress of St Andrew's Benn, a small girls' school in Rugby. She, it appeared, had heard of me through Miss Joan Enoch, my craft tutor, who had at one time taught in Warwickshire.

Miss Baxter's letter informed me that she was absolutely desperate – so desperate that she was willing to interview me to find out whether I could fill in, on a temporary basis, for one of her staff who had suddenly become ill. Unfortunately, she informed me, it might be difficult to arrange an interview, as she was going to visit relatives in London. It could not be mere coincidence that we were both to be in London at the same time. I lost no time in telephoning this possible rescuer, and we arranged to meet – in the waiting room at King's Cross station two days later.

I remember little about the interview, which is surprising, considering its unusual circumstances. I know that I decided to wear a bright yellow feathered hat. It seemed important that I must not give the impression that, because I was not able to see bright things, I was not concerned with them. I knew that in order to capture the attention of children I would need to be bright and vibrant, and these qualities were certainly embodied in that hat. It meant, too, that she could not possibly miss me in the crowd, and go on her way without our meeting.

Miss Baxter was a quiet lady, slow to reveal her own personality, but very perceptive and, as I soon discovered, yet another with a deep faith. She had to be. She agreed there and then to take me on half a term's trial, and promised to meet me at the station in Rugby two weeks later. She promised, too, that on returning from her holiday, she would make some enquiries about accommodation for me.

Two weeks after meeting Miss Baxter, on a Sunday evening in early September, I alighted from the train with two suitcases containing all my worldly possessions. My benefactress, true to her word, was there to meet me and invited me to stay at her home for that night, assuring me that she would make every attempt to contact, next day, a lady who could be counted upon to meet a challenge and who would in all probability be willing to take me in, if only temporarily.

Next morning I embarked upon my new career. We did not enter to a fanfare of trumpets. Clutching the right arm of the headmistress and trying to look nonchalant, as if I made that sort of entry into new situations every day of my life, I walked into the school playground. With the other hand, Miss Baxter steered an ancient bicycle, which well-trained girls relieved her of, stowing it away under cover. I followed my guide into school with what I hoped resembled stately dignity.

After introducing me to my form, Miss Baxter went about her business. The door closed behind her, and I was left alone with my class. I felt thirty-two pairs of eyes upon me. I could feel the questioning in those eyes – blind? How then? I felt too the sudden dawning of certain realization in some of them – *Wow, this should be good!* I must take an immediate stand.

I stood tall, managing to make my five feet three inches gain an extra half-inch, and delivered my first speech. 'Form 1B,' I said, in what I hoped was a tone of calm dignity and tremendous authority, 'Form 1B, you have been told that I am blind. What you have not been told, but I think you ought to know, is that I am not daft. It will be to your advantage to remember that, so I suggest that one or two of you take those silly smirks off your faces.' That was an inspired guess, and like a wave of electricity I felt their reaction. By the end of the first morning we all knew where we stood with each other. Fair play is a thing I rate very highly, and fair play on both sides. It did not take long for the girls in my class, and their teacher, to build up a healthy respect for one another.

I have always noticed that children, lacking the sophistication and self-consciousness we acquire when we become adults, adapt easily to unusual situations. When they are puzzled, they ask straightforward, to-the-point questions, and so long as the answers are straightforward and to the point, they accept those, too.

In a very short time, the children in my care gave very

little thought to my handicap. First and foremost, I was 'me', and the fact of my blindness no more important a part of me than that I had brown hair and blue-grey eyes. Sometimes, my apparent knowledge of all that took place in the classroom did puzzle them. There is a sort of electric feeling in the atmosphere when underhand things are going on. When I felt it, I would listen, and walk slowly, quietly, and apparently unconcerned, down the aisles between the desks. A tell-tale movement, probably not discernible to those who are not so reliant upon their sense of hearing, would give the show away. I would listen for the passage of the movement, and then pounce, closing my hand upon a folded note just being passed across the gangway. On one such occasion I took my booty to the staffroom at break. On one side was scrawled the question 'Do you think she can see?' And on the other 'I reckon so. She always knows what we're doing.'

My sense of smell, too, was instrumental in detecting school-girl misdemeanours. Red sweets, green sweets, yellow, or mint, all give off their own specific odour, and, when I invited offenders to deposit the offending object in the waste-bin, I was able to be specific as to its nature – a further cause for puzzled questioning.

Nor is it difficult to identify the sounds made by pencils being tapped, hair being combed, or comics being read under the desk. All of these things were tried, naturally enough, but the children soon realized that my original statement about the condition of my brain was not incorrect and, having had their 'try', they gave it up as a waste of time, and got on with the business of learning.

My own books, of course, were in Braille, and a blackboard was specially and simply adapted, with grooved lines on one side, and a grooved stave on the other, for use in music lessons. I was able to write fairly legibly – probably as legibly as some of my young students. As at college, the services of a retired teacher were offered, and gratefully accepted, and with her I would mark work in the evenings.

I knew I really had been accepted when the children began to bring photographs for me to look at. There were photographs of new babies, small brothers and sisters, themselves as bridesmaids, and numerous others. I would always take the picture in my hand, and invite its owner to describe it to me. After a while, I didn't even have to invite the description – it just naturally became a part of showing photographs to me.

True to her promise, before the end of that first day, Miss Baxter had managed to contact the lady she thought might be able to have me as a lodger. Mrs Fairlie seemed to have a taste for the unusual. She had lived in numerous different parts of the world, and had a great spirit of adventure. Her daughter had just got married, and her son had just started university. When my situation was put to her, she said that she would certainly put me up for a few nights, but that 'Dad' was away at the moment, and a more permanent arrangement would depend upon what he thought of me. Theirs was a lovely, homely family house that smelt of baking and was full of mementoes from their travels. My hostess was Scottish – a devout Presbyterian, who, I soon found, really lived her faith. I never knew her to turn anyone away, however much it might inconvenience her. She lived about a mile away from the school, and in the mornings I would be able to have a lift by car with a man whose shop was near the school, although I would have to make my own way back at night. I knew immediately that I could be happy in that house, and fervently hoped that when 'Dad' returned on Friday he would not disapprove of me. He loomed on the horizon of the week's end like a shadowy ogre.

Friday came and, at six o'clock, 'Dad' came too. No shadowy ogre this. He was one of the gentlest, most sensitive men I have ever known. There was no question of my being turned out on the streets. I was accepted and treated like one of the family.

They were happy years that I spent with those very dear people. Life was never dull in that household. 'Mum' was always involved in some project – mothers and babies, making toys out of things that others would throw away, picnics in the snow, visiting old ladies, and organizing functions at the church, of which 'Dad' was one of the elders. I especially remember the homeliness of Sundays. I would follow my own pursuits all day, and then present myself for a very special Sunday tea. A cloth would be placed over everything that was left from this feast, and I would be invited to accompany the family to evening service and usually did. On our return, the aforementioned cloth was removed, the wireless turned on and hymn books opened. During the half-hour of hymn singing on the wireless our little party around the table munched a bit, and sang a bit. It was a pleasant, safe time.

The path of life appeared, at last, to be smooth and easy. At half-term I was told that my appointment was permanent. I loved the work, and looked forward eagerly to every day. I had been accepted into a loving, warm family, and lived in a very pleasant house.

But there were some briars along that pathway, and more and more I felt them catching at me as I passed. At first it was possible to ignore them, but the wounds became more painful – in short, the old problem had returned. It was becoming more and more difficult to get around on my own. I still found it difficult to ask, 'Would you mind taking me to the dentist?' 'Could you spare time to go shopping with me on Saturday?' My colleagues were generous with their help, just as my fellow-students had been during college days. All the same, I did not cease to yearn for real independence.

Some of my pupils would walk part of the way home with me, but none of them lived as far from school as I, and the last half-mile was busy and noisy. When I was supposed to be marking books, I would be falling asleep through sheer exhaustion; my eyes would close and my head nod, in spite of my devising numerous strange sitting postures. It was as though life had become a treadmill. Thousands and thousands of steps had been taken, no energy spared, and yet here I was, back on the old spot I thought I had walked away from three years before –physical and mental exhaustion, angry frustration and bruised pride. What did it all mean? Had it all been a big mistake? How easy it is to become negative when the going gets tough.

It was then, just when I was becoming convinced I would be trapped there for ever, that the clouds once again parted and the sun shone through. It showed a fresh path, and I was filled with excited anticipation. A letter from the Guide Dogs for the Blind Association informed me that a dog considered to be suitable for me had been trained at Leamington Spa and I would have to spend a month there being trained to work with the dog. The dates given coincided exactly with the school holidays.

It was the beginning of a completely new life – a life of freedom that I had never known since becoming blind.

CHAPTER 5

Neana

And so it was that in April 1956, so many years ago, the old shoes of dependence and unsureness were cautiously cast aside to be replaced by slippers so light, they hardly touched the ground as I walked with a new confidence and a joyful, jaunty step into the years ahead.

Late one Friday evening I arrived for the first time at Edmondscote Manor, the guide dog training centre, in Leamington Spa. An Elizabethan manor house, it had been somewhat altered to accommodate dogs who were to be trained as guides for blind people. Training staff and guide dog owners who have been acquainted with the guide dog movement for less than twenty years would be amazed, I am sure, at the changes that have taken place during that period.

At that time the Association had hardly any breeding schemes of its own, and none of the dogs were 'puppy-walked'. Most of the dogs were bought from dealers, but when there was a shortage, as from time to time happened, trainers would go to local dogs' homes and even take in strays off the streets, provided they were of a suitable size and appeared to have an amenable nature. Many of the dogs were of a harder, tougher temperament than those to which, in more recent years, we have become accustomed. Now the majority are bred from known stock and spend their first year living with families who devote much time and patience to loving them and teaching them the basic obedience all puppies need to learn.

This meant, of course, that a higher percentage of the

dogs failed their training and had to be rejected. It meant, too, that the blind people who wished for the independence that these wonderful animals made possible must be very fit indeed; they had to be able to walk at an average speed of four miles an hour and any other handicap, however slight, would almost certainly prevent a person from being accepted for training.

I suspect that my first dog would have given my present one a supercilious glare if she had known about his air-conditioned kennel and comfortable dog-bed in my room. In her day, dogs in training were housed for the most part in converted stable blocks and during the month of training with their new blind owner they slept on the bottom of that unfortunate individual's bed. A person with long legs and a large dog was not likely to enjoy the luxury of uninterrupted nights.

In those days at Leamington students shared rooms in twos, so there was always a chance that one dog would be appreciably smaller than the other. If that were the case, and you were on good terms with your room mate, some arrangement could be reached whereby turns were taken to accommodate the heavier canine slumberer.

The seven training centres that the Association now has in Britain are spacious and, considering their purpose, very nicely furnished. Students have nothing to think of except learning to care for and work with the dog which has been carefully selected for them. In the fifties, Edmondscote Manor was shabbily but cosily furnished. In the one large room, which served as lounge, lecture-room and dining-room, a coal fire, protected by an old-fashioned nursery guard, burned brightly. Everyone, students, training staff and kennel staff sat around two large tables at mealtimes, and often the conversation included all present, regardless of the space between the tables. During my first month there,

one of the kennel maids celebrated her twenty-first
birthday, and the controller's son was christened: we all
joined in the festivities. After meals, students and staff
gravitated to the kitchen and helped with washing up. It
was truly like one big family, and great fun.

Each training centre has a resident guide dog owner.
Her roles nowadays are mainly those of receptionist and
secretary. The duties of Marjorie Radford, the wonderful, if slightly formidable, character who held that
position all those years ago were slightly more extensive.
When she was not answering the telephone or writing
Braille or typeprint letters, she could be found cutting up
pounds of meat for the dogs in training. After they had
been fed, she scoured out all the dog bowls with
dedicated vigour. However, as soon as we had each
acquired our dog, she handed the latter duty over to us,
making sure first of all that we 'made a proper job of it',
and then off she went to milk the goat so that the puppies
could be fed. I once asked Miss Radford what she did if
stray dogs made a nuisance of themselves. (At that time
all bitches were entire, and twice a year this made life
very difficult for blind owners.) She answered, 'Tell them
to clear off once and, if they don't, take off my dog's lead
and whack 'em with it, love.' I cannot imagine any
offending dog would ever come back for more.

The six of us who were to spend the next month together
were introduced to each other and to the trainers who
were now going to teach us how to handle our dogs, and
help us to win their affection so that they would want to
work for us with real willingness. A dog can only be
persuaded to do this very special work, it was explained,
if it is really willing to do it. Two apprentice trainers,
supervised by the centre's controller, were our patient
teachers. One of them, Brian Moody, still works for the

Association in a very senior position. We students were from all walks of life – three men and three women, I being the youngest.

I was almost at fever pitch with excitement, but just a little perplexed. Could it be that I had not come to the right sort of training establishment? This place was scrupulously clean, with no hint of a doggie smell. When I arrived there was not the smallest canine squeak or grunt to be heard. Well, it had been a long last day at school, and I felt I could leave the matter to be dealt with after a night's sleep. I was surprised and pleased to find myself sharing a room with a young woman whom I already knew vaguely, since she came from Cheltenham, my home town; we'd probably be able to sort out the mistake better together, if, indeed, there had been a mistake.

I awoke suddenly next morning. There had been no mistake, that was for sure. The air was full of noise – and a very particular brand of noise. Yelps, squeaks and excited barking did glorious battle with the dawn chorus, and won. 'Get down, Pip,' 'Leave Zara alone, Tina,' young voices yelled, and added to it all a percussion accompaniment on buckets and shovels. Six o'clock in the morning, and a guide dog training centre had burst into life with gusto.

After breakfast I rehearsed a few well-chosen phrases I felt sure would not fail to captivate the new doggie friend I expected to leap into my arms at any moment. I need not have bothered. As a now seasoned trainee, I reckon there can be few things less inspiring and more exasperating than that first day of 'work' at a guide dog training centre.

The lecture on animal behaviour, with snippets from the canine bible according to Liakhoff, seemed not unreasonable, although the relevance of the urinating

habits of bears left me somewhat mystified. The visit to
the doctor seemed fair enough, as did the rather dramatic
fire drill. I could hardly suppress my indignation, however, when one of the young men came in and
announced that for that day he was to be our dog, and if
we would kindly accompany him into the grounds, he
would endeavour to teach us how to give commands that
he was likely to obey.

We seemed to spend hours trundling up and down the
drive, tagging on to a harness-handle which he was
carrying, following it as he turned this way and that. As
each command to the dog is issued, there is an appropriate position for the feet and the body. Eventually it all
makes sense, but at that stage it seemed as though
everything had been designed for the express purpose of
causing the legs to tie themselves in an enormous knot,
leading eventually to the total collapse of the body.

And then there were those simple words like 'Sit',
'Forward', 'Right', 'Left', 'Back' and 'Stay'. At least, they
had always seemed simple enough before. I had never
realized that to utter them in a tone which would
eventually suit the sensibilities of a mere quadruped
would cause so much agony – and drama had been one of
my main subjects at college. Oh well, I came to the
conclusion they had to give these apprentices something
to keep them occupied while the hierarchy were too busy
with 'proper' jobs to keep an eye on them. Remembering
my own student days, I managed to think about it all
fairly positively, and went on managing to say 'Forward'
in what was considered an unsatisfactory tone for several
more hours.

Later that month, as I struggled to restore a little
circulation to completely numb feet and ankles, I felt sure
that the first two dogless nights must have been arranged
partly for humanitarian reasons, affording those who

were to become the proud possessors of seventy-pounders, or thereabouts, at least two nights of sound, unbroken sleep to build up reserves of strength for the hard labour of the month ahead – once it got under way.

At last the long-awaited moment arrived. After lunch the next day we were each told the name and breed of the dog to whom we were about to be introduced. Mine was Neana (pronounced Nina), a black labrador thirteen months old. (Nowadays, a dog of that age would hardly have begun the advanced stage of its training.) Then off we marched to one of the converted stable blocks, where each dog had its own separate 'stall' with a large iron gate, raised about a foot from the ground, to prevent it from getting out.

'Talk to your dog. It is important that it should come to know your voice,' was the parting stern instruction from the trainer as he left us for about ten minutes to become acquainted with our new friends. I poked my head cautiously through the space left by the open gate. A great wriggling bundle of legs, tail, dripping tongue and playfully nibbling teeth launched itself at me. Obviously an intelligent conversation would be out of the question for the time being. At least I could be polite and try to give a good impression to this long-awaited paragon who had attained almost god-like dimensions in my imagination over the months. 'Aren't you beautiful!' I remarked, rather lacking in original thought just then. That did it. The wriggling, wagging, nibbling and kissing stopped all in one go and, at that precise moment, this lovely, glossy youngster made up her mind, without even a second thought, exactly what she thought of me. From that day there was never any doubt about who was the boss of our outfit – and it wasn't me. It was delicately done, though, in utter good taste. No one but the most experienced student of the canine mind would have had the least suspicion that this poised, dignified animal, as she later became, masterminded our every movement from that day until the end of her working life.

From the first introduction, the blind student, under the watchful eye of experienced staff, is entirely responsible for feeding, grooming and exercising the dog whose affection and respect must be gained if the partnership is to be a successful one. This is absolutely essential if the 'unit' is to become safe and efficient in all circumstances.

Neana was obviously no more impressed with the delivery of my commands than her trainer had been, but at least I felt less self-conscious about asking, or telling, a dog to 'Sit' and 'Stay' than a young man. The main problem seemed to be that she and I always chose the identical spot to place our feet, which brought forth numerous long-suffering yelps from her, and rather ineffective apologies from me. So much stress had been laid upon the need to gain the dog's affection that I began to feel our relationship must be doomed from the start, for bruised paws and affection would hardly seem to be compatible. She did not, however, decline to accept the meal I offered at six o'clock, and when at ten o'clock that night I patted the foot of my bed and gave the instruction 'Up', no second invitation was needed.

It was then that I came to the conclusion that detachable feet would have made life a whole lot easier for the human race. Where on earth was I going to put mine at night? The problem was soon solved. My room-mate had been partnered with the smallest guide dog I have ever met, a little cross-bred creature with perhaps the vaguest hint of collie in her lineage. She proved to be one of the hardiest and most spirited guide dogs I have known, with lots of initiative but, for the time being, I felt her chief virtue lay in the fact that she was not a great solid labrador; we decided to take each dog in turns, thus being assured of reasonable alternate nights.

The training progressed in carefully graded stages. At first the trainer was always close at hand, actually holding the dog's leash for the first few days. We walked along quiet side roads, learning to follow the dog round natural and artificial obstacles placed at strategic positions by the trainer. Traffic work was gradually introduced, again on quiet side roads initially, mostly with cars driven by other members of the training staff. As a first-timer, I was astounded that, however much the trainer might try to entice the dog across the road, she stood her ground firmly while a vehicle was near, but the moment it moved off she obeyed the command to cross. When we went into the centre of town, I was amazed at how neatly we were able to weave our way through crowds of shoppers and completely ignore dogs, children playing with balls, or the noise of loud back-firing from vehicles.

One of the greatest hazards to blind people entrusting their lives to a guide dog is the unwelcome attention and nuisance value straying and unsupervised dogs can cause. I have had several very unpleasant experiences. Once, a very large, nasty-natured dog kept launching himself at my dog, making it impossible for her to walk, let alone ignore him, and I could not find a single person willing to help me. I do not think that would be the case nowadays, for the public is much more aware of guide dogs, and of the kind of help that is sometimes welcomed by their owners. On that occasion I was fortunate enough to be fairly near a telephone box, and, trembling from head to foot, kept ordering my dog to 'Find the telephone box.' Bless her, in spite of extreme difficulty, she obeyed, and at last we were safe. I dialled 999, and soon the miscreant was led away. Less dramatic, but potentially equally dangerous are the occasions when one is waiting to cross a busy road. Both dog and owner concentrate hard, wanting to judge just the right moment for the command 'Forward' to be given, and obeyed. Imagine how difficult this becomes if a straying dog, with nothing more pressing to do just then, starts prancing about yapping, and trying to play or fight.

These problems are partially alleviated by the fact that every prospective guide dog is positively discouraged from responding to other dogs while working. One that continues to be distracted by other dogs would quite definitely be rejected. Today the Association is able initially to be more selective and fewer dogs need to be rejected for dog distraction, but when I trained with Neana, there was a considerable number of dogs in kennels, waiting to be sold as pets. Once a month, these dogs actually earned their keep by assisting the class in training. Out they came, and were held on leashes by kennel staff at strategic points along each side of the drive. The young training staff referred to this as 'blood alley' and teased us at lunchtime as to the nature and size of the dogs we would encounter during the afternoon training session.

The idea was to give the 'Forward' command, and to walk straight down the centre of the drive, giving our own dogs a verbal correction each time we felt them showing any interest in the leaping, yelping mob. My dog passed with flying colours: she showed no signs of being dog distracted. However, I was told that, had I been the dog, I would have been rejected immediately and probably given away, having proved myself to be a very bad case. I had to agree. I had shuffled along, cringing behind my dog, and jumping like a prize firework every time I heard so much as a canine mutter.

It was thrilling as the month went by to feel the dog's affection gradually transferring from her trainer to me. It is absolutely essential that this should be so, and we were encouraged to spend as much time as possible with our dogs, grooming them, going over obedience exercises and generally learning to enjoy each other's company. Nevertheless, they never forget their trainers – all my dogs have made tremendous displays of recognition and affection when meeting them again many years later.

As the month went by the assignments we were set became more and more demanding and, although we were carefully supervised, we became gradually less aware of the trainer. He was obviously hovering somewhere in the middle distance, but only announced his presence if it was absolutely necessary.

I have always been stupid about traffic-light sequences. Just mention red, amber and green, and a big key turns in the lock. Each trainer whose unfortunate task it has been to acquaint me with this bit of road lore has started off with patience and optimism, but not one has cracked it, and each has had to admit defeat. On several occasions I have stood at a junction where the traffic is controlled by these incomprehensible monsters of this scientific age, trying to work out sequences, while the crowds around me have gone about their business, obviously unaware of my dilemma. I have secretly hoped that if I waited long enough my kind instructor would be moved by natural human compassion to rescue me. But no, not a single facial expression, either of panic, fear or 'damsel in distress', has worked, and in the end dog and I have had to sort it out ourselves.

This has usually meant that I have appealed to a passer-by with a less stony heart. In fact, this solution to problems is approved of and positively encouraged. Guide dogs are highly trained, wonderful animals, but in these days traffic conditions can be so dangerous that it is not fair always to put full responsibility on the dog, and at such times human help should be sought.

By the end of the four weeks' training we had been introduced to every conceivable situation we were likely to come across in everyday life. Country walks, city centres, shopping precincts, railway stations, free running for the dogs in parks – all were thoroughly taught and practised. We worked hard during that month, walking about eight miles each day, but we played hard too. We had many good times together. The training staff work six-and-a-half days a week during class, and then come back in the evenings to go with the students to the theatre, the pub, or a concert. I have always been amazed by their patience and kindness.

At the end of April, having said our farewells to all those dedicated people at the training centre, Neana and I stepped out through the gate – out on to a new path – a path of freedom. And so back to school the following Monday morning, but this time with no one holding my arm, no one to warn me of steps. I walked briskly across the playground with my new, trusty guide at my side.

From her very first day at school, Neana made it quite plain that I was no longer *really* in charge of Form 1B. Her large, brown, penetrating eyes left no one in any doubt about her thoughts and feelings. The first black mark scored by the class was registered at break-time, when the milk crate, containing exactly one bottle for each pupil, was brought in. Only a black dog could have given such black looks, and before many moments had elapsed the girls were putting contributions from their bottles into her empty dish. Ever after that, the crate held an extra bottle of milk, and that one was always given out first.

Neana also soon made it obvious that some of the musical efforts of the class left much to be desired. Actually, I could identify with some of her views: anyone who has had to listen to thirty-two recorders playing in disharmony has to admit that it isn't a pretty sound. As soon as the recorders were taken out of their boxes, Neana registered her feelings by sitting up in her bed, gazing heavenwards, and howling dismally. It was soon obvious that, on these occasions, life would be more comfortable for all if she were allowed to retire to the staffroom, where she toasted her toes by the fire, in more comfort than she deserved.

It was obvious, too, that the stories I read to the class during the last lesson each afternoon delighted her little more than the musical renderings. Although she never accompanied my reading with howls, she snored so loudly that the class was reduced to a giggling mass. Off to the staffroom she was sent. That dog really knew the right way to play her cards.

What a wonderful new experience, though, no longer to have to ask, 'Would you be able to take me to. . . ?' Although people had always been willing to help, I hated having to ask. Now I simply said, 'Fetch your lead, we're going to town.' I would then slip the harness around her and off we went, the new independence having almost the same effect as an intoxicating drink – it certainly went to my head. As time went by, many new words were added to the basic commands Neana had learned during her training days. It would be impossible to estimate how many words a guide dog comes to understand during its working life: in that respect, as well as in every other aspect of each dog's work and personality, there are marked variations. Dogs, like people, have their own particular gifts. At first we used only a limited number of shops in the town, but as our confidence increased, we added more and more places to our list. Neana's main confusion was between the wallpaper and newspaper shops, but since I made little use of either, that was not too serious.

The greatest problem about a trip to town with Neana was the fact that the café was one of the first places we had to pass. I say 'pass', but we never did. Try as hard as I might, I could never, by any method, prevent this new, determined friend of mine mounting the two steps and planting her bottom firmly on the top one. 'No, not today' had no effect whatsoever. This became extremely embarrassing, as very often a queue began to form. I could hear ladies asking each other whether or not they intended entering the café, and felt most conspicuous upon hearing the information being passed back along the line that they were 'waiting for the lady with the dog to clear the way'. Out of sheer self-defence I gave in, told Neana to 'Find a table', which she did, taking me to the side where there was an empty chair; then she curled up under the table, looking the epitome of the perfect guide dog. It was some time before I discovered that Neana had a close relationship going with one of the waitresses, and it had something to do with dropped sugar lumps – pure accidents, of course.

One evening, in the summer of 1958, I gave my first talk about guide dogs, more full of food than of confidence. Mrs Fairlie, refusing to accept my protestations that I was too nervous to eat the usual two-course meal she had prepared for me, more or less stood over me to ensure that every morsel was eaten. Imagine my horror when, arriving less than two hours later at the venue where I was to give the talk, I discovered that it was to be an after-dinner talk, and I was sitting beside the chairman, at the top table. I quake to think what those early talks must have been like, but I never ceased to be touched by the many kind and generous people I came to know through them.

Those were happy days. It would seem that I had everything I could desire: the profession to which I had no doubt I had been called, in a pleasant, easy school; a comfortable home with a delightful family; and many good friends. My social life was full. There were dances every Saturday night. It staggers me now when I remember how my friends and I would stand at the bus-stop in the middle of winter, dressed in scanty taffeta creations, ignoring goose-pimples the size of molehills, rather than cover our carefully planned splendour, which we had spent hours discussing the previous week. Stratford-upon-Avon and Coventry being so near, there were often trips to the theatre. And among my pleasantest memories are the picnics I shared with the Fairlies in the middle of winter, when we would dig holes in the snow, and put our cups of steaming soup and coffee in them to cool off.

However, the restlessness of youth and my increasing independence as I learned to put my trust in Neana had the effect that learning to fly must have upon young birds. I began to feel an urge to leave the safety of this nest and reach out to new challenges.

CHAPTER 6

Belper

At school we were joined by a new member of staff. Her recent marriage had necessitated her moving to Rugby from Belper, a small town in Derbyshire, and she talked nostalgically of the school in which she had taught there. It sounded progressive and exciting. There were more than five hundred pupils, both boys and girls. It had been built only two years previously, and had, for its time, remarkably good facilities. As we chatted, I felt I knew the staff, most of whom were very young, as well as if I had met them. That, I told myself, was where I wanted to be, more than any other place on earth.

My new friend took me at my word and wrote to the headmaster, telling him about me. No one was more shocked than I when my pipe-dream became a real possibility. Mr Parrott, the head of the school, was a man with a liking for the unusual, and who loved a challenge in whatever form it presented itself. What's more, it seemed more than coincidental that one of his staff had recently been advised by her doctor to give up teaching music, owing to recurring painful throat infections. I was invited by return of post to attend an interview for the vacancy, teaching mainly music and some English.

I remember sitting on the train to Derby, feeling almost grateful for the migraine which I knew would not exactly enhance my appearance, and would most certainly do little to help me seem intellectually bright. It was a humid day, and I arrived feeling sticky and consolingly drab – not at all the sort of person, I felt, who would fit into the set-up about which I'd heard so much.

But the moment I stepped through the door of the airy, modern building, I was overwhelmed by the warmth and friendliness of every single person I met. I immediately felt that I was being welcomed into a large new family and knew straight away that I wanted very much to be a part of it. Why couldn't the migraine and the sticky drabness have waited until tomorrow? Although the interview was held in the rather large, imposing library, the homely accent and direct, down-to-earth questions of those interviewing me put me completely at ease. One cup of coffee after leaving the library, I was told that the post was mine the following September, if I wished to accept it.

It was not without regrets that I said goodbye to Rugby, the school, my friends and the familiar haunts that summer. It was certainly not without some considerable trepidation that, just as three years before, I arrived one Sunday evening in September 1958 at the railway station of a town completely unfamiliar to me. This time, however, my faithful friend and eyes trotted beside me, glossy black tail waving, affording me the reassurance that I wouldn't be facing this part of the walk alone.

Once again, a delightful couple offered me hospitality. Not only do I remember Mr and Mrs Spencer's home for the kindness extended to both me and my dog, but equally I remember the evenings listening to music on the three-speed record-player my parents had given me for my twenty-first birthday. I learned there all I know about Schubert's *Lieder*. There, too, I was first introduced to the works of D. H. Lawrence, whom I regarded as an immensely romantic figure. And there I learned to speak the local dialect, 'almost as good as a native, for saying I was a foreigner'. It fascinated me. 'Ey up, Sorry,' was the most common greeting. I could never quite make out the reason for the 'sorry'. It is thought by some that it may have been a corruption of the Elizabethan 'Sirrah', a nice, old-fashioned explanation.

Belper, lying nine miles north of Derby, is a small town with an unusual mixture of industry and rural beauty. Even from the busy main shopping street, hills and fields are visible in all directions. The main road and the river run along the bottom of the valley, and from them the narrow roads run in all directions, sprawling in no particular order up the sides of the steep hills. Many of the houses are quaint and stone-built, although new housing estates have since sprung up around the perimeter.

There is a rough sweetness about the countryside with its foretaste of stone walls, mainly a feature of the more northern part of the county. As you cross side streets, gusts of wind unexpectedly laugh out at you, catching unceremoniously at your clothes and hair. The pavements seem to lie where they have been dropped. As I explored the routes I would need to know, I was often surprised when the pavement simply petered out, and if I did not wish to walk in the road, I would have to cross over to where another one started, for no apparent reason.

It was no easy task sorting out the geography of this odd little town with its unusual place-names, such as The Bone Mill, Walker Bottoms, Piggy Hill and The Clusters. I hardly dared even to ask for directions in case someone had been teasing me. However, a friend hit on the idea of making a map using spills and straws to mark the roads and this proved to be tremendously successful.

Soon Neana and I began to take the place in our stride – strides which became increasingly confident as the days and weeks passed. It was not long before she had sorted out the fact that the greengrocer's, butcher's and chemist's smelt just the same here as they had done in

Warwickshire and that two large, velvety brown eyes
could send out the message that a dog was ill-used and
undernourished, to anyone who cared to be taken in, just
as they had in our previous home.

The new school was both a challenge and a joy. It was
certainly harder work with mixed classes and, of course, I
had to start right from the beginning once more,
establishing a standard of discipline I found acceptable.
Again I adopted a mixture of listening hard to identify
sounds, following what my not inconsiderable intuition
told me, and acting on inspired guesses. Looking back,
one method I used for maintaining order seems rather
mean, but it worked. As before, I insisted that the pupils
sat in the places allocated by me, and I always placed girls
beside boys – that is, until they were in the fourth year,
by which time it would not have been a hardship.

As usual, I found children to be astonishingly adapt-
able and there was never a shortage of volunteers to help
me around the large building, carry the heavy Braille
volumes or groom the dog at lunchtime. That was
considered to be a very special privilege, much sought
after, and even had a marked effect upon the behaviour
of some of the less biddable characters. Neana was not in
the least impressed by her band of devoted admirers,
regarding them with the same disdain that she reserved
for most of the human race. On more than one occasion
she happily retrieved the ball thrown for her and kept
coming back for more, but if the ball happened to land in
a puddle or a patch of mud, she instantly deserted her
playmate and turned her back on anything which might
involve loss of dignity. She would return alone to the
staffroom and 'woof' at the door for admittance. Five
minutes later, a mud-splattered apologetic child would
knock timidly and return the ball. They always came back
for more.

I remember on one occasion sending a boy out of a lesson to stand in the hall because of some minor misdemeanour. After the lesson Neana spotted him standing obediently in his corner. She obviously considered that I had not reprimanded the boy sternly enough and, making it impossible for him to escape from his corner, told him in no uncertain terms what she thought of him. Judging by his remarks to a friend, overheard by the duty teacher, the poor lad was convinced I employed this black terror to keep miscreants in order.

That term the school had taken in a particularly large number of children; this meant that one teacher had no permanent base and had to teach in whichever room happened to be empty. I drew the short straw, as it were, and had to use five different rooms. Just imagine the strange procession at each lesson change. Neana, always dignified, marched at the head, trying to give the impression that she knew nothing at all about the rest of us. I came next, hoping I appeared completely in charge of everything. Then came the 'bearers' carrying my special blackboard with its stand, the gramophone, the box of records, recorders, books, and finally the dog's bed.

Many people find it difficult to approach a handicapped person, usually because of embarrassment rather than unkindness. The guide dog is a wonderful breaker-down of this barrier. A complete stranger spots the dog, and before he realizes what he is doing, has started asking questions about it, and the ice has been broken; he has discovered that a blind person is just like anyone else. My dogs have helped me to make friends with complete strangers on many occasions.

One evening, after a twenty-first birthday party at a

local pub, I bent down outside the main door, intending to put the dog's harness on. I suppose I was a little merry, and thought Neana was pretty merry too, as it appeared that her head was going round in circles. I ordered her to keep her head still, so that I could get the harness over it. An amused passer-by recommended that I should 'Try the other end.' Her tail wagged even more as I located the right end, and I had the satisfaction of knowing that one of us would steer a straight course home.

When I am asked, 'Where did you meet your husband?', my answer causes some surprise: 'He was on top of my dustbin.' But that is the actual truth.

After living with Mr and Mrs Spencer, who had allowed me to share their home for four years, I felt it was time I learned to stand on my own feet completely: I began to think about the possibility of having my own flat. Events then moved so quickly that I didn't even have to look for one. I was walking along the main shopping street with a friend one day, when Jean, who didn't even know that I had been thinking about moving, said, 'There's a flat to let over the electrical shop. Shall we go and have a look at it?'

Having nothing more pressing to do at the time, I agreed, and we were shown round there and then. I fell in love with it. A flight of stairs from street level rose to the first floor with its lounge, a doll's-house kitchen, and, for 1962, quite a glamorous bathroom. A quaint spiral staircase went up to two bedrooms. The small bedroom had an odd assortment of twisted chimney breasts, which formed funny little higgledy-piggledy alcoves. The building was very old, and I felt immediately that this little home had been sitting there, just waiting to put out a hand and catch me as I passed by. I knew that it was just the right place for me, and was even more certain when I was immediately accepted as the new tenant, even though I had no references.

Having agreed to the terms of tenancy, and signed all the appropriate papers, it suddenly occurred to me that I did not own a stick of furniture, and had no idea whatsoever about housekeeping. No sooner were these problems recognized, however, than they were solved. There was to be a sale of carpets and furniture at one of the local pubs later that week, and the bank manager agreed that my reputation was sufficiently good for him to risk allowing me a loan of a hundred pounds. The result of all this, and a visit to a second-hand shop in Derby, was one adequately – I would even go so far as to say tastefully –furnished flat. The only new items were a bed and one carpet.

My mother provided me with the few kitchen utensils I would need, and Jean offered to stay with me for two weeks, in which time she reckoned she would be able to initiate me into the not so gentle art of housekeeping. Soon my culinary efforts were adequate, if not always quite as tasteful as the décor. It was a lovely new game, which at that time I didn't need to play too seriously.

It was about that time that I discovered Mrs Rebecca Smith –later known as Mish. She used to clean the flat while I was at school and I associated her with the smell of polish and disinfectant that greeted me as I opened the door on 'her day'. It was lovely when, once or twice, I would get home before she had left, and she would stay and have a cup of tea with me. On those occasions I realized how much my parents' home meant to me, and how much I missed my Mum if I let myself think about it. That was years ago, but Mish still visits us most Mondays, bringing her pinafore and slippers so that she can help me out with various jobs around the house. She is one of those people who put enormous energy into supporting a cause from which they derive no personal benefit, except the satisfaction of helping others. A tireless fund-raiser for the Guide Dogs for the Blind Association, latterly she has served as secretary on the active and dedicated Derby and District Committee which co-ordinates the raising of thousands of pounds each year for the Association's work.

The flat even had a small garden – very handy for hanging out the washing, and running the dog. I soon taught Neana to take herself, last thing at night, across the tradesmen's yard and up a small entry into the garden, and to 'woof' at the street-door when she had sorted out her toileting for the night. During the seven years I lived there, this arrangement only misfired twice. On both occasions, although some years before she had had a hysterectomy operation following a serious illness, Neana believed herself to be in love with a shaggy dog who occasionally visited our locality. She must have met him on her way back from the garden and momentarily forgotten her loyalties to me. After a more than reason-able time lapse, with panic mounting inside me to fever pitch, I could only dial 999 and hope the police wouldn't be too put out about the nature of the emergency. Both times they obliged with alacrity and charm. I had, by that time, learned to make an exceedingly good cup of cocoa with which I rewarded them for their pains.

The owner of the shop, and of my flat, decided he needed to employ someone to help with his radio and television repairs. I soon became aware of the new occupant of the workshop across the yard, for he was often there until very late in the evening and never failed to greet me with somewhat saucy-sounding salutations. One day we actually met face to face at my dustbin.

I have always considered it a tribute to my standards of

hygiene that, on arriving with a pile of rubbish to be disposed of, the workshop 'voice' was actually there, body and all, sunning himself and using my dustbin as a perch. I remember asking him, somewhat snootily, 'Do you mind moving? This happens to be my rubbish bin, not a garden seat.' He obliged with his usual cheeky charm.

It was an unusual start to an easy, uncomplicated friendship. Ian fitted in going out with me between football and cricket, both of which he played for the village where he lived. I, too, had a very busy life, but always enjoyed the times we had together. He seemed to have no problem, right from the start, in accepting my blindness. In fact, it was he who always sorted out for me such things as a new cooker, or other similar equipment. He would read the instructions, get it straight in his own mind, and then show me, as though he'd known me all his life, the easiest way to cope.

It was Ian who showed me my first oak-apples, pulling the bough of the tree low enough for me to reach and touch their round, smooth surfaces; it was Ian who took my hand and guided my fingers around the beautifully formed nest of a jenny wren; it was he who, in simple sentences, described to me the half-hidden lake in the woods, with the old water-wheel nearby – the lake where, as a child, he had almost drowned. His direct, simply-told tale brought a great lump to my throat and heart for the little boy I could still recognize in this warm young man, so terrified of that water, and feeling its terror still. And it was on Ian's shoulder I put my head and sobbed as though my heart would break, after I had been told that my dear friend and constant companion would have to retire.

Neana had had her eleventh birthday and, as she got

older, it had been necessary for her to have several teeth extracted. One evening, while she was still rather dazed from the anaesthetic she had had earlier that day, someone rang my doorbell. Instinctively, and before I could stop her, she had struggled to her feet and, barking feebly, was half-way down the stairs, when her legs buckled beneath her, and she fell down the rest of the flight. We managed to carry her back to the sitting-room, and the next morning she seemed to be none the worse for the mishap: she readily pushed her head into the harness, and set off with me as usual for school.

I soon realized, though, that this tough, courageous creature was experiencing considerable pain with every step she took. That was the beginning of arthritis, which slowed her down so much that I don't think either of us really knew after that who was leading whom. We helped each other along, but both of us felt the strain. So, reluctantly, I accepted the expert advice of the guide dog trainer who came out to see her work and agreed that I would have to train as soon as possible with a new dog, when one became available.

My friend with the cheeky, boyish laugh was there, with gentle words of comfort – and that, although I would not have guessed it then, was not by any means to be the last crisis in my life when his would be the only comfort I desired.

CHAPTER 7

Dana

At the beginning of the next academic year, we were told that the school was to be visited later that term by Her Majesty's Inspectors. In those days that meant about a dozen rather formidable characters, or so they seemed to us, descending upon the school for a week, sitting in on any lessons, making copious notes, and producing a substantial written report some time later.

My teaching responsibilities had changed somewhat by this time. Although I still worked in the music department, and had complete responsibility for our school choir, I was spending more and more time with pupils who were then called the 'remedial' children – children who, for one reason or another, had learning difficulties.

For me, this soon became the most fulfilling work I had ever done. A very special bond grew up between these children and me. Not to be able to read fairly fluently by the age of thirteen is a considerable handicap, and the fact that I was handicapped, too, seemed to help them to gain the self-confidence less able children sometimes seem to lack. Some of them had so often been treated as failures by one person or another that they had come to think of themselves as failures, and so under-achieved even more. I knew the feeling: I had frequently had my own self-confidence dashed by the unthinking remarks of those I had to learn to excuse, because they didn't know any better. I had learned to battle against my blindness and the children, seeing this, were encouraged. They were not self-conscious with me, because together we laughed at the mistakes our differing handicaps caused us to make. I still meet many of them. Most of them are married and have children of their own now. We share affectionate memories of the past, such as the time when one of them, for a joke, got into the dog's bed. She took one look at the boy and, completely ignoring his presence there climbed in and curled up heavily on top of him. Shouts for help issued forth from under the dog's unresisting bulk.

That term I had a particularly large and lively class, and could only look forward to the visit from Her Majesty's Inspectors with absolute dread.

And then it came . . . the letter from the Guide Dogs for the Blind Association informing me that a suitable dog had been trained for me at the Leamington Spa centre. By this time poor old Neana was only just managing to hobble about, and had had two heart attacks into the bargain, so it was decided that I should have the required month's leave of absence. I dared to hope that I might miss the inspection, but soon discovered that I would return from Leamington on the Friday immediately before the dreaded Monday.

Off we went by car that Friday afternoon, the back seat piled high with the Braille books I would need to take with me to prepare some really impressive lessons during the breaks between training. Neana, that oh-so-familiar figure, who featured on every school photograph with me and who had attended countless school functions and outings with the class, was leaving school. No one could quite take it in, and there were some tear-filled eyes – not only those of the children.

We went by train to Birmingham, where my mother met us. We had decided that Neana should retire to my parents' home. They, like everyone who knew her, had always loved her and were only too happy for her to spend her last years with them. I shall never forget how difficult it was to speak as I bent down to unbuckle her harness for the last time. By now she was very portly, but still a real beauty to me. I squeezed her in my arms for a moment. 'Thanks, old girl,' I managed to whisper into her velvety black ear.

As I sat on the train which would take me on to Leamington, I would have seen little of the scenery, even if I had not been blind – my eyes were blinded with the tears which I couldn't suppress. Dear, dear old faithful friend. How much happiness and sadness we had shared. Perhaps the absence of words adds a deeper, more poignant dimension to a friendship with a dog. Ever-present, ever-watching, never forsaking, and never judging. Just loving, and here I was, rattling along, mile after mile further away. It was the first time I had ever felt I was abandoning a friend.

Neana spent three happy years with Mum and Dad, and died at the good old age of fourteen and a half.

The training centre was almost unrecognizable. Extensive alterations had been carried out, and now we had a very smart lounge, beautiful single bedrooms, and very up-to-the-minute facilities for the dogs, with smart hospital blocks and kitchens where the dogs' food was prepared that would have graced any modern home. The welcome was warm, and the six of us who were to train with new dogs soon got to know and like one another.

One thing that had not changed was that frustrating first day when we were all longing to know all about our new dogs: kennel staff and trainers alike had tightly buttoned lips, and not a morsel of information could be prised out of them. There were also the interminable marches around the grounds, trainer in harness, as it were, student issuing commands in hopefully authoritative tones and trying to adopt correct foot-positions to accompany each command.

And then came the magical moment, waiting all on edge in the bedroom, wondering how the meeting with the new friend who was to become my constant companion and eyes would go.

Dana, I was told, was a beautiful, rather small labrador. Her coat was a deep golden colour, and her chest and stomach pure white. She looked as though she wore frilly white pantaloons. Her large, soft eyes were rimmed with black, and she had, for a dog, very long eyelashes which she fluttered to good effect. She had the look of a bush baby, always rather surprised and wondering. This new little friend of mine would never put a foot wrong by choice. She lived to please everyone and immediately became devoted to me.

I must confess, however, that from very early days I felt that we were not ideally suited. This does not reflect in any way upon her work, which was almost faultless. I tend to be impatient by nature, and almost always in a hurry, probably because of a tendency to leave things until the last minute. After the month's training we returned home and straight into the great visitation. Try as I might, I always seemed to have only half the amount of time I needed in which to catch my bus. 'Oh, come along, Dana,' I would urge. She immediately assumed that I was not pleased, and would sit down, licking her lips apologetically. Not another step could she manage until I had crouched down beside her, put my arms around her quivering body, and explained that the fault was mine, not hers. That being understood and accepted, we would continue our 'run' to the terminus, usually to find the bus had just left.

Still, all in all the inspection went well. Her Majesty's Inspectors were not nearly as formidable as the picture I had conjured up, and as far as I was concerned, they had a number of helpful and constructive things to say.

As with Neana, Dana and I made many friends, and had many laughs too. There was the occasion when a friend went with me to the station one very sunny day. When my train came in, the porter grabbed Dana's leash from me and started to bundle her and my friend on to the train. I stood on the platform protesting that I needed to get on the train, not my friend, and in any case, it was my dog he had just helped himself to. He told me in reassuring tones that I had nothing to worry about and he would take good care of both of them. Just as the train began to move, my friend, recovering from the shock, pulled herself together, jumped off the train, and bundled me through the door, where I was reunited with a very worried Dana. I was so baffled by this episode that I rang my friend that night to see if she had unravelled the mystery. It appeared that, because of the bright day she had been wearing sunglasses, and the porter had assumed that she was blind, and that I had been there to see her safely aboard the train. On another train journey, I am not sure who suffered the greater degree of embarrassment when I put my hand out to stroke Dana's head, only to plant it caressingly upon the knee of the man sitting opposite. Covered with confusion, I apologized profusely and explained that my intention had been to stroke the dog's head. 'I've heard some excuses, but that's a new one on me,' he said.

A couple of years after having Dana, I began to feel restless. I had no idea why. I was enjoying my teaching and a couple of romances came and went fairly uneventfully. The restlessness took hold of me, and I knew that it was going to be something special. It was the same feeling I had always had when something new was going to happen, when I would have no choice but to be obedient to whatever was presented to me. And suddenly it was quite clear. For some completely unknown reason I felt the strongest urge to gain a qualification which would enable me to teach blind children. I had never thought that I would want to do this but, just as many years before, the feeling would not go away, and I could not ignore it.

After an interview at Birmingham University I was offered a place on the one-year course starting in autumn 1968. My own county agreed to second me on full pay for the duration of the course and kept my post at school open for me to return to the following year.

Lodgings within walking distance of the university were hard to find, but just before the start of term I was offered accommodation at Selly Oak. This would mean a half-hour walk along very busy, noisy streets, crossing a dual carriageway, and negotiating three sets of traffic lights. At that time Belper, which I now thought of as my 'home town', was still comparatively quiet and sleepy, and we did not have one set of traffic lights. A trainer from Leamington spent two half-days helping Dana and me to sort out the most urgently needed routes. My four-legged goddess took it all in and coped beautifully with the unfamiliar conditions. She weaved our way slowly and conscientiously through the crowds, and took the university campus in her stride. She blossomed under these conditions, and shed much of her shyness. I wondered if she was a repressed intellectual, as she seemed to prefer university to school life.

The move to Birmingham could not have been accomplished so easily without the help of Ian's Morris Minor van, which rolled up outside my new lodgings piled high from floor to roof with suitcases, books, bedding, pots and pans and, just to add a touch of the unusual, Dana, sitting in her bed which was wedged rather precariously among all the paraphernalia. I am not surprised that the lady who owned the house greeted us somewhat suspiciously. We must have borne a strong resemblance to a couple of tinkers. Having shown me how to use the antiquated gas cooker, initiated me into the art of feeding an indecently hungry electricity meter, and sorted out a piece of waste ground nearby, where I could exercise the dog, Ian clambered into his now empty van and chugged off into the distance.

I felt empty, too – horribly desolate and lonely. Whatever had possessed me? What on earth was I doing here? Much as I enjoyed all aspects of that year, the high spot of every week was Sunday afternoon, when the Morris Minor pulled into a lay-by across the road, and its owner and I spent the next six hours companionably chatting, laughing, walking in the Lickey Hills with Dana frisking around, asking for a ball to be thrown, or even at the launderette. Our relationship felt as comfortable and easy – and as necessary – as breathing in and out. We never discussed the future, and I didn't even think about it, but I could not imagine being without that sensitive, reassuring friend of mine.

I was the only blind student on the course and had a rather unfair advantage in that everyone else had to discover the mysteries of Braille. It was just as well, though, for I soon discovered that my brain did not work as quickly as it had fourteen years before. We were a light-hearted crowd, on the whole, and didn't need too much excuse to have a party or go ice-skating or ten-pin bowling.

The course included a considerable amount of practical work, and we spent half a day each week teaching in schools for visually handicapped children. The classes were small, with seldom more than a dozen children in them. It was both challenging and rewarding work, and I enjoyed it enormously. There was the added bonus for me that the children used Braille, so I could mark work without any assistance. Yet I knew, but knew not why, that I could never settle to teaching permanently in a school for the visually handicapped. So what was I doing here? I knew deep down that the riddle would be solved some day. I had not been able to run away from that persistent inner call a year before.

It had been an interesting, stimulating and rewarding year, but it was good to return home to my little flat and walk the familiar paths, climb the steep hills and hear again the rugged accent of the people I now thought of as 'my folk'.

Buying a small house of my very own at the top of a steep, winding road seemed to be a necessary gesture of independence. Once again, the Morris Minor came into its own as removal van, and the smaller items were transferred in the cars of various friends who, with a great air of industry, and in carnival mood, soon got the little house looking more or less like home. I loved that little house, and spent hours and hours dreaming of how I would alter, furnish and decorate it, and the larger part of my salary turning those dreams into realities.

There was hardly a day when I did not see Ian, and then, at the end of October, we decided that it was time we thought about getting married. He bought me a beautiful ring with an oval ruby surrounded by diamonds. I used to hold up the finger on which I wore it, and imagine how those stones would be sparkling, and hope that everyone would see them catching the light as I moved my hand. We had known each other for six years, and had enjoyed a deep, warm, uncomplicated friendship, but Ian told me long afterwards that he had waited until he was quite certain that what he felt was love, not pity because of my blindness, or admiration for the way he felt I coped with it.

We were married the following Easter Monday, 12 April 1971, when the buds on the trees were just bursting into pale fresh life and the daffodils were proclaiming by their brightness that it was time for all nature to wake up and start merrymaking. On the way to church I cried with a joy I felt so deep down that only tears could express it. The church was very full and I felt proud as my own school choir preceded me up the aisle. One of them sang an anthem with a recurring refrain: 'See that ye love one another'. Her bright young voice rang so purely through the large church that, even as I signed the register, I had to stop and listen, my heart full to overflowing with the wonder of beautiful things. How appropriate that on this Easter Monday morning our new life began.

CHAPTER 8

Married Life

After our honeymoon in Stratford-upon-Avon and the Cotswolds, I returned to school, where life went on as usual except that I had a new name.

How I wished that my efficiency in the classroom could extend into my kitchen duties. It must have been fairly obvious to the most uninitiated observer that my culinary experience was limited. Trying hard to impress, I triumphantly marched across the kitchen on our first Sunday at home, bearing aloft, with what I hoped would be an air of nonchalant familiarity, a pan of sausages, bacon and mushrooms. Before I had got half-way to the breakfast bar, unknown to me, I had tipped the pan at a rakish angle, and sausages and bacon rolled around the floor at such a rate one could have been excused for thinking they were practising for the Olympic Games. I burst into tears, utterly deflated and humiliated. 'Never mind,' my new husband comforted, 'your floors are clean enough to eat off.' I thought he was making fun and renewed my lamentations with even more force.

The following week I became very adventurous and prepared boeuf stroganof. I left it simmering while I took a wifely interest in the roses in the front garden. I hadn't checked the definition of 'simmer' and once or twice wrinkled my nose and gave voice to my thoughts on people who have bonfires on Sundays. On going back to put a light under the rice and stir the beef, I was faced by a pan full of something that felt like cinders and smelt atrocious – remarkably like the bonfire which had so offended me. It took two weeks to get the saucepan clean.

Stewing rhubarb for an hour didn't do much for the second of our set of three new saucepans. It was a long time before I learnt to laugh at my mistakes, and I certainly wouldn't have thanked Ian, at that time, if he had done so. Gradually, over the months I improved, and was thankful that my husband kept insisting that he enjoyed ordinary plain food.

In December 1971, at about the time that we learned that our first baby was on the way, we left our little house at the top of the hill and moved to a larger one further down. Here we began to make our first real home together.

During that year, we dug up floors and took down walls and chimney breasts. The coal fires that had seemed so cheery when tended by the previous occupants, could manage only a sulky-looking blackness for me. The dear, elderly gentleman next door, who was later to be known as Grandad and who involved himself in all our alterations, commented, 'You only seem to be able to mend the fire out, lass.' I had to admit that there were other things I could 'mend' more efficiently, and so the dejected black holes were replaced by gas fires.

Our neighbours on both sides became wonderful friends, and coping with the baby, when he arrived, would have been a far more daunting experience without them. Meanwhile, I continued teaching until twelve weeks before the baby's birth. I must say those last weeks at school exhausted me, especially as he was born in August, and it was a hot summer. It was with very mixed feelings that I said goodbye to my colleagues and pupils at half-term. I knew I would miss them all very much. School life had really been all the life I had ever known.

However, I had much to do preparing for the baby. People had been so generous. A number of mums had knitted sweet little garments. Often in the afternoons I would take them all out of the drawer and imagine the little body that would soon be inside them.

August the seventeenth was a very hot day. For some reason I cried as I left the house to go to the hospital. I knew that I had come to the end of a chapter in my life and was nervous about turning to the next page. But once we were at the hospital, things began to happen so quickly that there was no time to think about such things – I just had to get on with the job in hand. Ian spent the whole day with me and, between the awful pains, I could think of nothing except his packed lunch of potted-meat sandwiches, which he'd left in the car. I was certain that lack of refrigeration would cause them to poison him. At seven-thirty, just as 'Top of the Pops' was finishing, our baby son was born. He looked incredibly solemn and wise. The nurse who delivered him said she was certain he was prime-minister material. With the instinctive doting love of a mother, I was sure that she was right.

The staff in the hospital prepared me well for when I would no longer be able to call on them for help. Disposable nappies were used generally, but they fished out some old, conventional terry-towelling ones so that I could get used to changing Adam without sticking safety-pins into him. They initiated me into the art of baby bathing and were so helpful in every way that at the end of ten days I was reasonably confident with him. Adam was a contented baby and, when I became very ill with an abscess, at the age of five weeks he accepted a bottle as though he had never known anything else.

As long as I was very methodical, there were seldom any hitches, and my neighbours were always only too willing to help. As time went by, the most problematic task was spoon-feeding. I would sit the wriggling little scrap with his back to me, and place my forefinger under his bottom lip. Having loaded the spoon with food, I would proceed to aim for the mouth. Just at the point of arrival, the little head would spin round, jerking the food all over the place or receiving it in one of his ears. To allow for spillages, I had to make half as much food again as he needed. Then I hit on the idea of inviting friends to lunch, and suggested they might enjoy feeding the baby while I put the finishing touches to our meal.

As the baby grew into a toddler, and then into a small boy, there were fresh delights. I remember teaching him his colours. I stuck gummed coloured paper on to card, and Brailled each one with its name. We used to turn the pages, saying the name of each colour. I took particular pains to speak to him in a visual way, picking him up to watch the 'big red bus' coming up the hill. As he went around the house playing, he gave a running commentary on everything he was doing. This was very helpful to me. A friend helped me to make story-books by cutting up printed versions and sticking them on to Braille paper. We then wrote the text in Braille, so that I could read the story while Adam looked at the pictures. We had much fun with an electronic ball which buzzed whenever the stopper was pulled out of it. One day we lost the stopper, and that was not such fun.

One day, while I was hanging nappies on the line in the garden, I was suddenly overwhelmed by a feeling of panic I had never experienced before. I left the washing basket by the line and rushed indoors. As the weeks went by, this dreadful panic attacked me more and more often, until I could hardly bear to go out of the house alone. It was a ghastly, hopeless feeling. I could have been so happy with my husband, baby and friends, but the big hostile world seemed to crouch menacingly outside the door and filled me with awful fear. Together Dana and I hid inside the house from this fearful creature, the world. I was certain that I would never go out alone again. The thought depressed me, for Adam would not always need so much attention and what on earth would I do, cooped up indoors for the rest of my life?

It dawned upon me that I had become a prey to that dreadful sickness agoraphobia – a fear of the outside world. It lurked like a great, dark monster behind every innocent-looking bush and wall. It crouched behind trees and around corners. It peered menacingly, waiting for me around every bend, just waiting for the moment to pounce, black and dreadful, all claws and teeth. When it came, I would have no way of escape. I would not be able to run. My legs would try to run, but be incapable of movement. My heart would race for action, but my limbs would be immobilized by clutching, clawing fear. Oh God, was I to be condemned to a life of hiding away from the world and all its beauties? I must break out and fight against this awful, silent beast which threatened to consume me.

Each month, a lady called with a catalogue from which I ordered cosmetics and perfume. I have always loved to experiment with make-up, having, of course, to rely upon a friend to help me choose colours. I have been lucky to have friends who shared this interest and would give advice, which is absolutely necessary when one is not able to have the reassuring help of a mirror. One month, the lady with the catalogue told me that she would not be calling again, as she was taking up a full-time job. I was taken aback when she suggested that I might like to take over her job with the cosmetics firm. My pride would not allow me to tell her about the beast that waited outside for me. I accepted her offer, hoping that before the area supervisor came to sign me on, I would have thought up a good excuse for changing my mind.

Soon after, one of my former pupils came to see the baby, and just to make conversation I told her what had happened. Without hesitation she said that she would help me. She was not old enough to do the job herself, but she'd love to go round the area with me. It looked as though there was no escape route, so in due time my young friend and I started on our rounds.

I was dismayed by how much confidence I had lost during those months of being practically house-bound, and felt at first as though I would never again be able to make even tolerably intelligent conversation with adults. As the weeks went by, however, the challenge got into my blood and I began to look forward to the evenings when we went knocking on doors with our catalogues. The people we went to were friendly and welcoming. It was good, too, to have some pin-money to fritter away on luxuries. I don't remember for how long I did this little job, but I had to give up eventually because a hard winter with deep snow made it too difficult to get around.

I was not allowed to vegetate for long, however. One afternoon there was a knock on my door. The complete stranger sounded so pleasant that I invited her in. She told me that she had heard I raised money for the Guide Dogs for the Blind Association. Thinking she was going to offer me a donation, I confirmed this information. She then went on to explain that she worked for a firm manufacturing plastic kitchen containers, among other items, and asked me if I would like to invite a few friends along for a cup of coffee one evening, and she would come and demonstrate her wares for them. I would be given commission on the amount she sold, and for a charity this would be paid at a higher rate. I could hardly refuse.

In the event, I enjoyed the occasion, and went to similar parties at the homes of my friends. I must say, though, that the last thing I expected was to be asked to become a demonstrator myself. However, that was what happened, and as I was missing the pin-money I had earned with the cosmetics firm, I felt there was no harm in giving it a try. Again, the challenge urged me on. I was fascinated by the different methods one could use to show the full potential of the different items. There was something reminiscent of my days in the classroom, and I looked forward to each booking. My friends must have been very long-suffering and probably still have cupboards full of all sorts of things they have long since forgotten how to use. We had lots of fun at these parties, but I knew that this was only a stopgap.

Winter came round again, and with it a bleakness inside me. I had to admit that although I could face the beast outside the house when I was with other people, the fear that gripped me if I tried to venture out alone was overwhelming. During the outings the parties provided, I was able to push it into the back of my mind, but on winter afternoons, shut in the house with a toddler and my ageing dog, who was herself becoming increasingly nervous and dependent on me – *me*! – for support, I brooded on my situation, and became horribly depressed and inward-looking. Oh God, I moaned again, what is it all about? What purpose is there? I loved my husband and little boy. We had a pleasant, comfortable home – but I didn't want to be a prisoner in it for the rest of my life.

Just when I thought I could go on no longer, and yet could see no way out, the telephone rang. I was surprised to be asked if it was true that I had a supplementary certificate for teaching visually handicapped children. I said that was so, thinking that, since I had never used it in a practical way, I was going to be asked to pay back the year's salary I had received while doing the course at Birmingham.

But what I did hear coming down the telephone was so exciting that I thought I must be hallucinating. The friendly voice told me of a boy who had lost his sight as the result of an illness. He was not well enough to attend a residential school for the blind, but needed a home teacher with the special qualifications I had. I could hardly take it in. Someone really needed me. I held back, though, and explained that I had a toddler and no means of transport. That was no problem I was told, since the boy's mother would be willing to bring her son to me. The authorities would provide everything I needed, and I would be paid according to the hours I worked.

We turned our spare bedroom into a classroom, and within a week I had met my new pupil. Gary came to my home most afternoons when he was well enough, and my heart warmed to him from the very first day. In spite of devastating health problems, this courageous child put every ounce of effort that he could into all he did. For him, many of the things that a normally healthy child would not have to think twice about doing demanded an enormous amount of perseverance. But eventually our lessons had to stop, when a recurrence of his illness made it necessary for him to go into hospital. The news of his death some months later made me more sad than words can tell.

What of the little golden goddess during these months? From early days I had been aware of her suspicion of children. She tolerated the children at school and in fact even grew to like them as she came to realize that they loved her. Anyway, she knew she could hide in the shelter of my authority over them. At home I always warned friends with small children that, while I trusted Dana implicitly, for I knew her to have a gentle, loving nature, I also knew that she would say very rude things to their offspring if they ventured too near. Having made this clear, I felt it was then their responsibility to ensure that a safe distance was kept and Dana's domain not encroached upon. This always worked well.

When I first took Adam home from the hospital, I remembered having read somewhere of a woman who had had a possessive labrador and who, on taking her baby into the house for the first time, had encouraged the dog to sniff the feet of the new arrival. Following this example, after Dana had greeted me profusely, I told her all about the new member of the family, explaining that I hoped they would treat each other with great respect. Then I proffered the ten-day-old toes and stuck them right under her wet nose. She did not even bother to sniff. Ignoring the proudly held bundle with which I was trying to acquaint her, she came and lay as close to my side as she possibly could without unseating the baby.

And that was her way from then on, whatever we were doing. She attended bathtime, feeding time, changing time, and later story time, sitting not even a hair's breadth away from me, but completely ignoring the presence of the new member of the family. If I unwittingly shut her out of the bathroom it was not long before I heard the sliding door being pushed open by her nose, and there she was, as close as could be, but with an air of 'I'm not really here at all, and I don't want to know what that thing is that you're dipping into that water.'

As Adam learnt to crawl, and later to walk, mutual respect grew of its own accord. If he crawled towards her, Dana would utter one deep, throaty growl, and he, completely unimpressed, would turn in his tracks and address not another word or glance in her direction. I knew he adored her by the way he spoke of her and watched for her when she went into the garden. That the feeling was mutual was proved by Dana's restlessness when my elderly neighbours invited Adam round to watch 'Play School' and have tea with them. Every time she heard his voice through the adjoining wall, Dana would prick up her ears and whine gently until his return.

Since both Dana and I had more or less completely taken to the house at this time, she needed exercise that I found myself unable to give her. She had always loved and trusted Ian, and actually made a point of letting him, rather than me, know if she was feeling under the weather. He loved taking her out on her leash in the evenings, and she did need the exercise. However, although she started off excitedly enough, as soon as she could no longer see the house, she turned smartly round, and Ian had no choice but to follow her home. During those days she was only happy if she could see me and be with me. What a pair we were.

I received a letter informing me that a trainer would be coming from the Bolton guide dog training centre to carry out a routine visit. These visits take place about once a year so that any difficulties of which one may not be aware can be spotted and sorted out. Both owner and dog can develop bad habits in the work and these can be quickly dealt with and expert advice given.

I dreaded the arrival of this unknown visitor. Our area had been transferred to the care of the Bolton centre several years earlier, and I knew the staff only through the names on correspondence. The young man, whose name I cannot remember, took one look at Dana and summed up the situation. Veterinary reports showed that tranquillizers had been prescribed during the last year.

Then the awful moment came. He said that he'd like to watch us at work – *outside*! I began to make all sorts of excuses. My small boy kept me confined to the house rather a lot, and we hadn't been able to work much lately; it had been a dreadful winter with a lot of snow, and no one but a fool would have ventured out in such conditions. And so on, and so on. There was a long silence. This young man was far more astute than I had given him credit for. 'I think in view of Dana's age, it would be wise for us to retire her and train a new dog for you,' was the gist of what he said. That was it. Confession time had arrived.

Dreadfully ashamed, I began to pour the truth out to him, all the fear and tension and panic. I did not believe that, even if I went through with the training, I could ever again venture into the great, frightening outside. My mind flashed back to those days in my late teens and early twenties when I had taken enormous risks to maintain my independence. I recalled those first days with Neana and the sheer bliss of walking out with her, knowing that I was perfectly safe. I remembered the thrill I felt when we stepped out at such a confident speed that we overtook other pedestrians. I thought with gratitude and pleasure of the freedom Dana had given me in the busiest thoroughfares of Birmingham and of how, on several occasions, this quiet, patient creature had even guided me safely in London. Could this be the same me, trembling at the mere thought of everything that lay beyond my front gate? It was not that I in any way mistrusted the capabilities of the dog that would help me to regain the independence that had once been life itself to me. It was that great, lowering beast called open spaces.

I tried to explain all this without revealing too much of my inner dilemma to the kind man with the hint of a north-country accent. After listening quietly, he advised me without any display of emotion to talk to my doctor and tell him that I 'wanted' to be independent again. That was it. Was there the tiniest suggestion that I had been holding on jealously to this fear? Well, if so, I'd show him that that was not the case.

Within a few weeks I had been referred to a specialist who had made a special study of phobias, their causes and treatment. I visited him once a week and soon began to feel the benefit of the treatment, which amounted to little more than learning to relax completely, and talk my way, step by step, through the anxiety-making situation. Within four months I had informed the controller of the Bolton centre that I felt I would be able to use a guide dog in a limited sort of way, if they felt that they could find one that would be able to cope if I began to panic. A month later, the head trainer rang to tell me that a dog had been found which they were certain would meet my requirements. I was horrified when he said that, if handled well, the sky would be this dog's limit. Was he really placing such a responsibility on someone who would do well to handle her own problems, let alone help a dog to attain its full potential? I felt that I must give it a chance, though, and agreed to attend the course which would be held during the month of August.

I shall never forget the last time I attended the hospital in Derby for my treatment. Afterwards, Ian and I took Adam and Dana to a park. I remember sitting on a roundabout with Adam, and he called to Dana delightedly each time we went round past her. It was a lovely warm, sunny afternoon. We called at a café for our tea before going home to give Dana hers. She refused to eat it, and a little later was violently sick. I was not worried, as I had had similar experiences with her through the years, and put it down to her nerves. I became very concerned, however, when the same thing happened the next day. We took her to the vet and were told to give her a light diet of fish, chicken or rabbit, and three doses of medicine a day.

She refused everything I offered her, and the sickness became worse. We were, by now, visiting the vet almost daily. The poor dog was noticeably thinner, and Ian said her face looked very drawn. I tried to entice her with tit-bits from my hand. Out of love for me the dear little soul tried to eat, but choked on the food and was unable to swallow it. She managed to drink small amounts of water with glucose.

One day the vet took Ian to one side and had a muttered conversation with him. That night, Ian had the unenviable task of telling me that there was little chance of Dana's getting better, and that the vet feared she was very ill indeed. I refused to believe this, and said that it was only a matter of time and perseverance. I had seen her like this before, and I knew that the tide would turn soon. What I did not know, and what everyone found so difficult to put into words, was that if I had been able to see her, I would have been in no doubt about the truth of what they were trying to tell me. The whites of the poor dog's eyes were very yellow, her coat staring, and her once pretty, golden face very pinched and drawn.

One night I started to go upstairs to bed. As usual, she pattered behind me, but very feebly indeed. Half-way upstairs I was aware of a strange sound – she was trying to drag herself up on her stomach. She had not the energy to climb the stairs, but her loyalty prevailed over her weakness. If only men and women were as loyal to those they love. Utterly devastated, and horribly ashamed, I went back downstairs, and spent the night on the settee, with my hand all the time on my poor little friend, just to make sure that she was still breathing.

Next morning we phoned the vet, who agreed to come and put her out of her pain in our home. That morning she greeted the milkman with a feeble bark, which she had not managed for several mornings. It was just as though she was saying goodbye to him. I did not dare move far from her, because she was so distressed if she lost sight of me. Ian came home at lunchtime and a friend took Adam out for the afternoon.

When the vet came I suddenly lost my nerve and asked Ian to stay with her. I waited at the top of the stairs. All of a sudden, I thought of this lovely creature who had been my companion for ten years, through days of laughter and days of tears, and who had never left my side, however afraid she may have been. I was ashamed and ran downstairs, hoping I would not be too late. I knelt on the sitting-room floor. There was a bowl of fragrant-smelling roses on the dresser, breathing their perfume into the air. I knelt with the poor little thin body across my knees.

The vet was so kind and sensitive, telling me everything she was doing. She gave the first injection, and the light body in my arms relaxed. As the second needle went into her leg, my dear, dear Dana quivered, sighed, and left me. Her body was wrapped in the blanket on which she had always lain, and she was taken to the surgery for a post-mortem to be carried out. I was told the next day that she had sclerosis of the liver, a complaint from which she could not have recovered.

CHAPTER 9

Martin

I felt conspicuously overdressed as I stepped out of the train at Manchester railway station. A friend's wedding could not be missed that morning, and there had been no time to change. A silk leopardskin-look dress and ridiculously high-heeled shoes, in which I could hardly balance let alone walk, must, I had to admit, have looked totally inappropriate to the guide dog trainer who was going to drive me the last stage of the journey to Bolton. I was to spend the next four weeks there learning to handle the dog which, if its credentials were anything to go by, might be expected to sprout wings at any time. Miss Woolrich, the young woman who greeted me, only just managed to hide her incredulity. It was not, she told me later, outside the bounds of possibility that somebody who dressed up like this for a train journey might appear for training sessions similarly decked out. The thought of the eight miles a day walking in those high heels would have caused the stoutest heart to sink.

Adam was now three years old and both sets of grandparents and several friends had offered to look after him during the day while Ian was at work. I had no fears about his needs not being provided for. We had explained the situation to him, and he seemed to accept it all quite happily, knowing that his Daddy would bring him to see me each Sunday, that there would be picnics each week and a brand new dog when I came home.

The Bolton training centre had an invitingly homely smell. I was surprised that there were twelve of us in the class – four women and eight men. As the days went by, and personalities unfolded, I felt that I had rarely known such a cheerful, talented crowd. One of the men could play just anything on the piano, and we invented our own words – usually about the training staff and each other – and put them to popular tunes. That month was, in the main, full of laughter and sunshine.

Our dogs had been trained by three apprentice trainers, under the watchful eye of the head trainer. Miss Woolrich was one of them, and it was not long before I put two and two together and came to the conclusion that she had trained the dog I was to have. I made sure that she could not miss the fact that my feet were now shod in extremely sensible, flat, lace-up shoes.

Of course, there were the inevitable trips round and round the grounds, coaxing the trainer 'Forward' and commanding her to 'Sit', 'Stay' and urging her to go 'Right', 'Left' and 'Back'. And then came the magic moment when all twelve of us sat in the students' lounge awaiting the great revelation with bated breath. I heard the names of various students being announced, and then the information about the dog which they would soon be meeting. My name was almost at the bottom of the list and I could hardly contain my excitement, tinged, however, with a fair amount of apprehension. And there it was at last, my name being called: 'Mrs Taylor, your dog's name is Martin. He is a cross between a labrador and a golden retriever.' The look of horror on my face was all too obvious.

'What on earth is the matter?' Miss Woolrich asked me.

'A dog?' I gasped. 'Called Martin? What a name for a dog. And a cross? I didn't think you used mongrels.'

The loaded silence that followed this unfortunate speech made me realize that I had lost, in the space of time it had taken to make it, any approval the flat shoes may have gained for me. In a voice as calm as she could make it, this young woman, whom I had already gathered was utterly devoted to every dog she trained, informed me that a first cross and a mongrel are two completely different things. The Association had only very recently started using this particular cross which was of their own breeding, and they had very high hopes for its success. 'Actually,' she went on to inform me, 'we like his name, and think it suits him.'

Dreadfully embarrassed, I tried to excuse my blunder, and only got myself into deeper water. 'It's not that, so much,' I explained. 'I just didn't realize it would be a male. I mean, they have really rather dirty habits, don't they?'

That was too much for the poor young woman. Utterly lost for words, she left it to her boss to explain in a cool, level voice, 'None of the dogs we train have dirty habits, Mrs Taylor.'

'No, of course not. I wasn't thinking. I'm sorry.'

Miss Woolrich recognized my confusion and her heart melted. 'Watch him,' she warned, meaning the dog, 'he likes handbags.' Oh well, if the sky was his limit, who could deny this paragon of the canine world the odd handbag or two on his journey there?

I sat in my room, waiting for the patter of the handbag-snatcher's feet to announce his arrival. A lawnmower chose that moment to splutter into action just outside my window, so that the first thing of which I was aware was an enormous furry presence in the room.

'Hello,' I ventured by way of impressing him with my flair for making conversation. But eloquence was not needed to bring out the natural showman in this fellow. Just that one word, and his front paws were on my shoulders, and he was covering my face and neck with doggie kisses. I soon learned that he liked perfume, too.

Then he caught sight of himself in the mirror and, being typical of his sex, lost no time in rushing over to have a better look at his handsome face. Then he must have caught sight of my slippers, for he bounded across, caught them up in his mouth, made a circuit of the room and grabbed my purse the second time round.

Eventually I caught him, and relieved him of my belongings. He stood still then, and I ran my hands over his domed head, long silky ears, strong broad shoulders. His coat was soft as down, and his thick, bushy tail never stopped wagging. I had been told that he was the colour of ivory and had beautiful dark eyes and a black nose. I thought I had never encountered such a lovely dog, and knew immediately that I loved him. I felt instinctively that this dog and I would be absolutely right for each other.

That night Martin settled down on his bed, wagging his tail from time to time to remind me that he was there. I put the light out before getting undressed. I felt vaguely embarrassed having a male watching me so closely, albeit a canine male.

Ian still speaks with wistful nostalgia of his first encounter with this lovely animal whose great dark eyes seem to draw like a magnet even those who would not normally look twice at a dog. As he and Adam came round the sweep of the drive and stopped the car, Martin and I were standing outside the french window of the students' lounge. Ian was amazed at the size of the dog beside me – he actually weighed ten pounds more than Dana. As my husband walked towards us, Adam trotting excitedly at his side, Martin became beautifully alert, pricking up his ears. This changed the whole expression of his sweet, soft face, and Ian felt immediately that this dog he did not know had accepted them as part of me and would be willing to give them his love and loyalty, too.

* * *

Most dogs happily accept kennel life, enjoying the rough-and-tumble play with others of their kind. Martin was one of the odd few who cannot cope with the competitiveness of the pack situation. During the day, when most of the dogs were having a great time together in the spacious run, he would sit miserably by the wire fencing, looking for all the world as though he would burst into tears if someone didn't rescue him soon. Sensitive to the differing needs of all the dogs in their care, the training staff do not leave such dogs to 'sit it out'. Often they are taken under the wing of one of the kennel staff, and spend the time when they are not actually being trained in the house.

Miss Woolrich frequently took dogs for whom she was responsible home with her at weekends and so there was nothing exceptional about the fact that his was a familiar face in her parents' home. I think he must have watched attentively the tricks she taught her pet dog Nero, for I soon found that Martin would 'speak' on command, and without a command if he got on the wrong side of the door. He still loves to 'give a paw', and counts it an honour to be asked to 'die for your country'.

One thing was causing me some concern, but it was of a delicate nature, and I didn't know how to broach the subject. However, after about a week, seeing how well the partnership seemed to be growing, Miss Woolrich asked me what I thought of him now. I told her that I had already become very attached to the dog, and felt instinctively that we would become a successful working unit. That would soften the blow that was to follow. I was still not entirely happy about his being a male, for in spite of her reassurances on the first evening, occasionally when I was sitting down Martin would back up to me and lift one hind leg on to my knee.

'What happens then?' she asked me, with a smile in her voice.

As I See It

'Nothing,' I told her. 'I don't give him a chance. I push him down as quickly as I can.'

She laughed and laughed until tears rolled down her face. I thought there was no accounting for warped senses of humour. Managing to gather herself together at last, she said, 'I forgot to warn you about that. He must have been cuddled a lot as a puppy, and hasn't realized that he's grown so big. He still tries to get as much of himself as possible on your lap, if you let him. Mind you, that isn't much these days.'

Having sorted out that slight worry, I acknowledged that this gentle giant possessed all the qualities I could possibly have hoped for in a dog.

That happy month went by quickly and, although I was longing to get home to my family, I was sad to leave everyone. During the month I had felt my confidence growing daily, not least because of Martin's complete indifference to the other dogs and his air of solemn wisdom. He never seemed to get agitated, and on the odd occasions when the old panic did grip me, he sat beside me, serene and unruffled. My fear evaporated under his calming influence.

Adam now went to play school three mornings a week, so Martin and I could go out regularly. As we stepped out confidently, overtaking most other pedestrians, I found it hard to believe that less than a year before I had resigned myself to a bleak future in which independence would play no part. I had quite forgotten the sweet taste of freedom, the intoxication of facing a challenge, and the thrill of stepping out into the unknown. Where had the fearsome beast gone? Where was it lurking? I did not know, and I did not care. I was free, free, free, and never again was I going to allow those prison doors to close on me. I stood and listened to the larks singing in the fields and the water cascading over the weir. I marched along the main road with lorries roaring by. I trod completely unknown paths and explored unfamiliar ways. Sometimes the enemy, fear, would try to step out into my path, but with my trusty new friend trotting confidently alongside me I would push the foe aside and never look back to see whether or not he had gone.

Now I had a new pupil, Nadeem, coming to me every morning. Although he had a little sight, he had to do all his lessons in Braille. Nadeem was very bright, and in a one-to-one situation I found this demanding, challenging work. This lasted for only one term, after which he was transferred to a residential school for visually handicapped children.

Immediately, though, home tuition was required for Barbara, who could not settle in a residential school. She, too, came each morning. Teaching basic skills, such as reading, writing and number, is as natural to me as breathing, but I felt that there was something more that I ought to be offering this teenage girl. Although I could in no way describe myself as being naturally domesticated – sweat, tears and mistakes had been my foremost teachers – I set myself the task of teaching Barbara what I knew of the mysteries of housekeeping. I felt that I would be eminently qualified for this, as I had learned so much through my own errors.

For I had not forgotten the occasion when Ian called to me on his way out to work that he had picked some peas from our garden, and they were shelled and ready to cook. I had made a liver casserole that day. Eager as ever to employ any method that would save on washing up, I grabbed from the fridge the container of what sounded like peas when I shook them and tipped them confidently into the casserole. Ian always dished up the meals, mainly for the sake of speed. (On occasions my sense of humour has evaporated if someone has come to the kitchen door and caught him at this. 'What do you think of the meal I've cooked?' he would ask them, twinkling, to tease me. I always rose to the bait.) On this occasion, removing the lid from the casserole dish, there was a stunned silence from my husband's direction. 'What's the matter?' I asked, thinking he must have burned himself. 'It's just that I've never seen a purple liver casserole before,' he said. He soon realized that he had forgotten to tell me that he had stripped the blackcurrant bush, whose fruit he had also put into the fridge. I felt that all was not lost. Many exotic recipes use meat and fruit together, and this one would be full of vitamin C. However, one cautious taste convinced me that the last thing I needed that day was vitamin C. I was mortified when even the dog refused it.

On another occasion I was making a cake. I lined up the ingredients rather hurriedly, because I could hear Adam playing happily on the stairs. I wasn't in the mood for having a toddler up to the armpits in cake mixture just then, so planned to get it done quickly and in peace. It was to be a ginger cake, and we like them hot. I mixed all the dry ingredients, and added the eggs. Opening the drum of ginger, I heaped the teaspoon as high as I could. Just then, little footsteps came trotting along the hall, and a voice calling, 'What are you doing, Mummy?' 'Nothing,' I lied, taking in a quick breath that, just in time, revealed the smell of curry powder, which happens to be packed in the same shaped drum as ginger.

Well, there were two tips, probably obvious to most, but not to me, until learnt the hard way: check all ingredients by smelling them before use and wherever possible label them in Braille.

But I never learned my own lesson completely. Only a few weeks before my first eye operation I made a cup of coffee. Thinking I had a sachet of cream which I hadn't used in a restaurant, I squeezed the thick liquid into my cup, turning my nose up at the common or garden milk my father-in-law was offering me. The coffee, when stirred, frothed in a most spectacular way. Licking the 'cream' from the spoon, I discovered that shampoo does not enhance the flavour of coffee.

Each blind housewife, and blind man for that matter, will find their own methods for coping in the home, in just the same way as those who can see choose the ways that suit them best. I use very few gadgets, mainly because I am rather good at losing the small ones and find it a bother to assemble the larger ones. A Braille thermostat on my cooker, a measuring jug with raised lines at each quarter of a pint, a potato peeler and egg separator which, in fact, can be bought in any shop, are my main gadgets. I have had others, but after playing with them for a while, they seemed to find their way into the back of a cupboard.

The domestic task I found most difficult was vacuuming, as my vacuum cleaner seems to have a voracious appetite, and however carefully I checked the floor beforehand, it would find numerous small objects to gobble up. Peeling potatoes was also, for me, tedious and time-consuming, although a serrated knife makes scraping new potatoes easier, as you can feel where the knife has been. When vegetables come to the boil, the bubbling can be heard, and if there are other noises in the kitchen, the vibration of the saucepan handle gives the same information. There are few jobs in the home which a blind person is not able to do as well as a sighted counterpart, but everything takes much more time and greater concentration, and one has to be very organized.

Barbara and I stuck to simple dishes, such as crumbles, scones, shepherd's pie. We did not weigh our ingredients, but instead used the tablespoon method. A heaped tablespoon of flour and a flat tablespoon of the heavier ingredients, such as sugar, weigh roughly one ounce. The eight-ounce block of margarine is cut into halves or quarters, diagonally, according to the amount required. That was the way I worked. Others will have their own methods.

We had great fun during these sessions, and learned, through them, far more than simply cookery. The best part of it, though, was the immense sense of satisfaction when a dish was produced that could be taken home for the rest of the family to try. Working with this young girl gave me tremendous satisfaction. It was both challenging and rewarding. Now, too, I was able to understand why I had felt compelled to become qualified to teach the visually handicapped. At that time there was no other person in Derbyshire with that particular qualification.

Not being domesticated hadn't really mattered until I was married. Cleaning and washing were things I had never needed to know about. During the years at the flat, and later at the little house at the top of the hill, housekeeping almost seemed like a game, with something safe and nostalgic about it. The smell of lavender polish and soapsuds and the 'clonking' sound the scrubbing brush made, as Mum applied it vigorously to the front doorstep, were a part of the timelessness of childhood, and came pleasantly back to me as I washed and polished windows and dusted and arranged ornaments. These tasks had a somewhat therapeutic effect, too, and the physical exertion seemed to clear my mind and enable me to find more inspiring and exciting ideas for school the next week.

As wife and mother, however, I became almost obsessive about housework. I washed all the upstairs paintwork one week, and downstairs the next; I cleaned and polished curtain-rails at least once a month, and sometimes even polished the lavatory seat and the taps. I seemed to think that by so doing, I would in some way prove to my family that I really did love them. I derived no personal pleasure from these tasks, but I was prepared to do this for them, because I loved them. They were singularly unimpressed by my self-imposed and, I now realize, rather silly martyrdom. I am sure that if they had come home and found the beds not made and the dishes unwashed they would not have noticed, so long as they could smell something appetizing in the oven for tea.

Someone said one day, 'Your husband must be a very good man, taking you on, the way you are.' That really stung; it hurt deep down, right inside, and kept coming back to me, even though I knew it was only a careless remark, not intended to hurt. With renewed vigour I attacked the tiniest sticky mark on furniture and paintwork, running my fingertips over any surface where dirt or dust might lurk, and attacked every tiniest crease that might dare to try to defy me on newly washed clothes. I was determined that no one should ever have the opportunity to think that my house or family were untidy because I was blind. I drove myself ridiculously hard at that time. I didn't want my offspring to feel different or deprived because of me. What a dreadful waste of energy and time.

A number of my friends make their own bread. The air in their kitchens is heavy with the sweet aroma of golden crustiness, with its message of devotion and efficiency. Visiting their houses, I would discreetly zip up the top of my shopping bag to hide the wrapper which would tell all these amazons of the culinary arts that I fed my family on slices of pappy plastic bread. At last I felt shamed into equipping myself with a large bowl and joined, twice a week, the band of pummellers and kneaders. Now *my* kitchen smelt homely and welcoming, and *my* neat rows of loaves smiled up at visitors as they came through the back door.

I felt full of virtue as we munched our way through the thick, coarse slices, happy in the knowledge that I was laying good foundations for my family's future health. Deep down inside, though, I admitted to myself that I loathed the pummelling and kneading sessions. It all took hours, and I would much rather have spent the time playing the piano, or reading, or visiting friends. What a relief it was therefore when, by first one and then another carefully worded remark, it was made quite clear to me that my menfolk preferred slices of pappy plastic bread, and were willing to take a chance on their future well-being.

Gradually I came to realize that all this preoccupation with cleanliness and tidiness and striving after perfection were not so much expressions of love and care for my family as a way of satisfying my own rather foolish pride. What did it matter if one or two people did think Ian had taken on a lot? We all take on a lot when we get married, whatever our circumstances, and probably become bigger and better people as, through the years, we offer our individual gifts to the partnership. Ian discovered that he actually likes 'messing about' in the kitchen. He makes good jam and, when we invite friends round for a meal, he gets on with cooking it, quietly and efficiently, whereas I flap and snap at everyone who has the nerve to venture anywhere near the kitchen.

On the other hand, I am good at making up stories, dreaming up ideas for projects at school, helping with English essays. This arrangement suits us all. Everyone groans, almost audibly, when they become aware that I am launching into one of my periods of intense domestication. It is a sign that I am overtired and likely to be unreasonable and explosive.

When Adam was a toddler and Ben was on the way a social worker came to see me. I couldn't believe my good fortune when she said that she would arrange for someone to come for two hours each week to help me with the cleaning. I am immensely grateful to her and to the ladies who, through the years, have made the house sparkle from top to bottom, all in the space of two hours.

CHAPTER 10

Miracles?

It was in late 1976 that Ian and I discussed the possibility of having another child. Adam was four and would soon be going to school. I felt that I had not got babies out of my system and as Barbara's sixteenth birthday was fast approaching she would only be with me for a little longer.

The specialist I consulted was not optimistic about my becoming pregnant at 41, but confirmed that there should be no danger to myself. He warned us, of course, of the increased possibility of an older mother having a baby who might be handicapped. Three months later we knew that Adam would not be an only child for much longer. He started school two terms before the baby was born.

It was the tenth week of my pregnancy. The air was cold and clammy and the familiar sounds of traffic were slightly muffled. Martin and I walked into town and I had soon filled the shopping bag. It was heavy, but no more so than usual. Suddenly it began to snow heavily: I must get home before the pavements became too treacherous. Martin and I always moved at speed, but that afternoon we ran most of the way up the steepish hill. When I got in I was completely exhausted. By the time Adam came in from school, the snow had come down in some style. It had banked up against the front door, and I had to lift him in over it. We sat together by the fire watching 'Play School' on the television. As we sat there, I was gripped by dreadful pain and I realized that something was very wrong with the baby. Telling Adam to sit still and not touch the fire, I phoned first Ian and then the doctor, explaining the symptoms. Then I got into bed. The doctor was pessimistic, and felt that I should be taken into hospital as soon as possible. I wanted to stay at home in the secure environment with which I was familiar, and promised to stay as still as possible and to ring again immediately if things got worse. That night neither of us slept. I prayed as I had not prayed for years, pleading for the life of my unborn child. Some time in the early hours I suddenly felt an incredible peace and knew that all would be well. When the doctor came next day, he was amazed that I had not had to call him in the night. Less than a week later all was completely normal again, and life went on as usual. That was when I began to believe in miracles.

The rest of the pregnancy was completely normal. I continued to go out with Martin until exactly one week before the baby was born. Martin seemed completely unperturbed by the fact that I was two-and-a-half stones heavier and that my normally fast, light footsteps had become a heavy plod.

My one dread was that when the baby arrived I would be confined to the house again. My neighbours, who had helped out so much with Adam, were now very elderly and not at all well. Having regained my freedom and rebuilt my confidence with the help of my completely dependable dog, I was anxious not to lose it again. I talked to the health visitor about this worry, and she promised to speak to some women from St Peter's, the big parish church. They had formed a group whose aim was to help people who experienced difficulties of one kind or another. Soon she was able to tell me that they were willing to help, and would visit me after the baby's birth. Everything was sorted out now, and it remained only for the baby to arrive.

Benjamin was born on the eighth of July. When Ian saw him, he laughed and laughed and said that he looked like a garden gnome. I thought him very beautiful. Again, I could not speak too highly of the sensitive attitude of the hospital staff.

When Ben was about six weeks old, I was visited one afternoon by a pleasant young woman from the church group to tell me that she and one or two of her friends were willing to help me out with minding the baby. Now Martin and I were outward bound again – and Ben, carry-cot piled high with sterilizer, nappies and a list of instructions so that there was only just room for him, went off for the morning about three times a week.

Everyone loves to visit a new baby in the neighbourhood, and so of course there was a steady stream of callers. I looked forward to having a chat and a cup of coffee with them – and probably somewhere in the back of my mind was the thought that some day soon a little help with spoonfeeding would not go amiss. I remember one day having three visitors. They all admired the dark-haired little chap in the pram, but I sensed an uneasiness in each one, as though she was wanting to tell me something, but didn't know how to put it. I checked the nappy, and made sure, too, that he had not been sick. Assuming I must have imagined it, I covered him again with the cotton sheet and left him to sleep. When Ian came home, he peeped into the pram. 'How long has Ben been helping with the washing-up?' was his first question. My mother had once given me some very large tea-towels. They were white, and a wide green stripe down the centre actually bore the legend in bold print 'TEA TOWEL'. Oh well, it had done him no harm, and its message has certainly not rubbed off into his psychic depths – or has it? He manages to leave the kitchen at top speed even now, if a tea-towel is handed to him. An essential ingredient in the personality of a handicapped person must be a sense of humour.

One of my new friends from the church asked if I would like to go to the family service one Sunday. She told me that there was a crèche for the babies and provision was made for the young children. She also offered to pick me up in her car. Thinking it would seem ungracious to refuse, when they were doing so much to help me, I agreed to go along. Although I had never stopped believing in the God who seemed to have been around and fairly close to me for most of my life, it was many years since I had taken part in any sort of organized religion. But if I put the joint in the oven and made a pudding before I went, I knew that Ian wouldn't mind seeing to the vegetables. Actually, it was the church where we had been married and so, in a way, I always thought of it as 'my church'.

The congregation was large, and I had never before come across so many children in church. I was struck by the warm friendliness of everyone there. The service was in modern language, and there was a pleasant blend of the traditional music on which I had been brought up and new, catchy songs, accompanied by guitars, flutes and percussion instruments. Afterwards, over a cup of coffee, I was introduced to such a lot of folk, all chatting away like a large family. I agreed to go again the following Sunday, and the following one. Oh dear, had they assumed that I would become a regular? I didn't think I wanted that to happen, but perhaps if I just kept going until Ben started play school, they wouldn't notice if my attendance dropped off. Just at present, though, I must let them see that I really was grateful for all their help – and in any case, I was beginning to know one or two of them really well, and enjoyed their friendship for its own sake.

* * *

For us, 1978 was an eventful year. Ian's mother died rather suddenly a month before Ben's first birthday. She was always such a laughing person and knew just what to do in any situation. We missed her very much.

Then in August we moved house. I only went out of curiosity 'to look' at the house round the corner, in what the estate agents described as a 'desirable residential area'. It was detached and larger than our house, with magnificent views, I was told, at the back. In the valley, as I can see now, the river twinkles in the sunlight and the mill stands out proudly against the skyline. The whole town sprawls lazily up and up the hills on the other side of the valley, and to the right the countryside climbs away into the distance, carrying in its arms the stone walls and farmhouses typical of this area. As the house is built into a steep hillside, it has two storeys at the front, but at the back there is another floor underneath the living-room and kitchen, so that there are two flights of steps down to the patio and another to the garden.

One or two people knew I was interested in the house, and immediately felt it their duty to warn me how eminently unsuitable it would be for a totally blind woman with two children. How would I ever have a moment's peace with all those steep steps? And how difficult it would be for me to cope with such tasks as hanging out the washing.

That was it! I must have that house to live in – I could not resist the challenge. That was more than nine years ago: I have learnt more sense since. Nowadays my comfort would take first place, and probably pride would not even get a look-in. Most of us mellow with time.

We moved in, and it *was* hard work. The view was magnificent, though, and I always felt drawn to its loveliness, even though to me it was invisible. I would stand for ages on a summer's night just breathing in the aura of its beauty.

In the late autumn, I could tell that Martin was losing weight rather rapidly, and then other people began to remark on it. When I first had him, a pancreatic deficiency had been diagnosed, but tablets kept him stabilized. We increased the dose, but the weight loss continued. He did not play as much, and slowed down a little in general. Tests were carried out, and the vet was not happy about him. There was a possibility that his pancreas was in serious trouble. I was advised to exercise him as little as possible and inform the Guide Dogs Association immediately. His case was serious enough for tests to be arranged at the veterinary research department at Liverpool University. Unfortunately, it would be closed over Christmas and would not reopen until after the New Year.

It was not a very joyous Christmas for us. We didn't tell Adam, of course. We loved this patient, sweet-tempered creature so much. Everyone loved him. He was known by name all over the town: wherever we went, people often wished him 'Good morning' and totally ignored me. Surely this patient, gentle lifeline and friend was not going to be snatched away from me so soon?

I had heard some of the people at church, which I still attended regularly, talking about prayers for healing. I knew that some of them met fortnightly and prayed for sick and handicapped people. Ready to try anything that might help Martin not to die, I rang one of them, feeling rather silly as I asked, 'Would you consider praying for a dog?' I was amazed at the reply. 'Why not?' she said, in a matter-of-fact voice. 'They are God's creatures.' I told her all about his problems, and a group set about praying for Martin with as much devotion as they would have done for a sick child. There had been no mistaking the desperate fear in my voice.

As soon as the university department reopened, Martin was taken there by a trainer. It was very cold and snowy and, as I said goodbye to him, I felt as bleak as the January day. I was told that I would be contacted as soon as there was anything to report, but that I could ring any evening to find out how the dog had settled. That week seemed to have far more than seven days in it. I was astonished at the cheerful voice at the other end of the phone telling me that she was the head kennel-maid at the Bolton training centre. 'Yes?' I could find no words to frame the question I was afraid to ask. 'The tests have all been done. We'll bring Martin back to you on Monday, if that's all right.' 'But what's wrong with him?' I had to ask now. 'They can't find anything wrong,' she told me. 'It's like a miracle, isn't it?'

Martin began to regain the weight he had lost and we resumed our very active life together. Later we travelled all over the county, after I started to give regular talks about the work of the Guide Dogs for the Blind Association, and the demands of my growing children involved us in many activities. Martin has now celebrated his fifteenth birthday and has had no medication for six years.

CHAPTER 11

Plateau Land

It was when I found myself responsible for the children's choir at church that I realized there was a class-teacher inside me just longing to be let out again.

In spite of the more informal type of service I had now become used to, we still had a traditional, robed choir, who were mostly children. At times there were as few as five, at others as many as twenty. When it looked as though the choir might cease to function, I allowed myself to be persuaded into taking it on for about six months. Through the six or seven years that I did actually take the wheel, I was helped by a number of adults who didn't mind helping to maintain the vehicle, but didn't want to drive it.

I am sure that there never was such an unorthodox church choir. Oh yes, the children were robed, but they somewhat resembled a scene from St Trinian's as they ambled or skipped, according to individual taste, in what I fondly liked to term the 'procession'. No one in the congregation batted an eyelid if one of my songbirds waved to a pal in the back row. It was plain from the start that we were going to rise to no great heights of perfection with the rendering of classical anthems or Anglican chant. Over the years I did manage to slip in the odd serious item when they were off-guard, but we concentrated in the main on light, catchy songs.

Choir practice started with prayers and a short talk, usually given by me, which was intended to lift the soul above earthly thoughts. In fact, I rather suspect that the pious attentiveness served as a cover-up for disposing of chewing gum and disgusting-smelling sweets, or an unflattering, mimed discussion of my shoes or some other, to a mere adult's mind, irrelevant matter. After about an hour of more or less singing, there was a completely crazy twenty minutes when we played riotously noisy games. I say 'we' but I usually took shelter behind the piano at these times and left my more physically courageous friends to direct operations. We finished with drinks and biscuits, which to the unsuspecting passer-by might excusably have been taken for a mouth-cramming competition.

At one time, I decided to have an introit sung from the back of church, immediately before the first hymn. To add to its effectiveness, I asked that this should not be announced. There would be a note from the organist to quieten the congregation, and, I considered, the music which followed would lift their thoughts above earthly things. Having run out of suitable material for this purpose, I lit upon the idea of encouraging the children to write their own simple words and fit them to well-known tunes. For the beginning of the Easter service one year, I suggested the tune of 'London's Burning'. We could sing it as a round, so that a few words could be made to go quite a long way. I chose as eminently suitable the words submitted by a ten-year-old, the first two lines of which went, 'Christ is risen, Christ is risen; he is here, he is here'. We practised it on the Monday before Easter Sunday, and I was really pleased with the way it sounded, and congratulated myself on my own brain-wave.

On the day itself I gave copious instructions as usual and stood, with my little brood around me, at the back of the church. The organist gave the first note, I counted 'One, two', and took a deep breath, hoping to set a good example for my choristers. Completely horrified, I suddenly became aware that I was singing different words from my young charges. Although I changed them immediately, it had been noticed that the Easter service that year had commenced with an announcement by some of the choir, that 'London's burning, Christ has risen'.

For all that, on most major festivals and quite often on ordinary Sundays, the children produced some quite lovely contributions which never failed to delight their listeners and caused me to forgive all and turn up again for choir practice the following Monday. Apart from everything else, this group served to keep me in touch with the changing attitude of youngsters towards adults. I would not have missed those six years, with all their frustrations and real joys.

When Ben started school, the house seemed empty and quiet. Martin and I increasingly made visits to schools, giving talks about the work of the Guide Dogs for the Blind Association and trying to give children an insight into the lives of handicapped people. I so much wanted to preach the gospel that handicapped people are just people who, because of their disabilities, may have to adapt their ways of doing things.

I wanted to get over the message that handicapped people prefer sympathetic understanding to pity and that, in fact, pity is a negative, destructive emotion. I felt, and still feel, that all young people need to be encouraged to communicate with handicapped people, and so learn to think of the person first, and the handicap as having little more significance than baldness or a big nose. I myself have so often been crushed and demoralized by the 'Does she take sugar?' attitude that still exists among people whose very last wish would be to cause hurt.

As present-day policies will mean that more and more

disabled people will be living in the community, I feel
that these opportunities to put the message over are
invaluable. Over the years I have received dozens of
letters from schoolchildren which have shown how
receptive they are. These letters, and the drawings that
usually accompany them, have never ceased to delight
my family and me.

This work, along with that with the choir, made me
more and more aware of the steady knock, knock, knock
that was going on inside.

I was often asked questions, after a talk, which related
specifically to my attitude to my blindness. My answer to
the inevitable 'Would you like to be able to see?' was a
truthful 'I suppose every blind person would like to be
able to see.' To the question 'Do you mind not being able
to see?' I again truthfully replied, 'No, not most of the
time.'

I honestly felt that in all the major matters of my life my
handicap made little difference. It was often an irritation
to me when, for instance, I dropped something which
rolled and I could not find it immediately. It was
frustrating if I planned to match a pair of tights with a
particular outfit and forgot to ask one of the family to
check them before they all went out. And on wet days I
envy people who drive around in warm cars, arriving at
their destinations dry and respectable, while I get wet
and bedraggled and resemble, at times, something the
dog has dragged from under a bush, rather than his
owner. But such minor irritations are surmountable, and
not worth getting into a stew about. I have no time for
bitterness. None of us knows what is going on inside
another person. One does not have to be handicapped to
have a broken heart or a hurt mind.

On the other hand, most handicapped people would
agree, I am sure, that there are times when they are made

to feel less than whole. People rarely mean to be unkind. Indeed, it is often their very sensitivity which makes them unable to cope with a situation they do not understand. An unexpected encounter can embarrass them, so that they neither think nor act quickly enough. This is when a sense of humour comes into its own, and can gently make a point. Once I got on to a bus in an unfamiliar area. Preferring to sit just inside the door, as there is plenty of room for the dog there, I asked if the seat was empty and received no answer. As I lowered my bottom to sit down, it made contact with the ample lap of a passenger who had been so nonplussed by my needing to ask whether or not she was actually there – most people couldn't miss her – that she had been rendered speechless. Smiling as pleasantly as I could, I remarked, 'Didn't you notice me? Good thing I'm no heavier and wasn't wearing spiked knickers.' Immediately she laughed, and we chatted for the rest of the journey.

Again, I needed my sense of humour one day when I was waiting at a request bus-stop. As I heard the 'whoosh' of air brakes, I raised my hand to attract the driver's attention. The vehicle came to a halt a short distance away, so I assumed something was preventing it from pulling right up to the bus-stop. 'Forward,' I urged the dog, but he refused to move. 'Forward,' I commanded a second time. 'Find the bus.' Again he stood solid as a rock. 'Come on, don't be silly. We're getting on the bus,' I told him, trying not to sound irritable, and waving my arm in the direction of the rumbling engine. Then I began to think dark thoughts about all those stupid people on that bus looking at my fruitless efforts to budge my dog, who must either have stepped in glue or momentarily lost his hearing. Why on earth didn't one of them just get out and offer a bit of help?

I was surprised to hear the door on the driver's side open: I didn't know they had a door of their own. A very tall man came over to me, put an immense hand under my armpit and, before I knew what was happening, I was lifted bodily from the ground. My legs made walking movements, which felt at least two inches above ground level.

Dragging the poor dog behind me, for I had no choice, I was propelled in this undignified manner across a very wide and busy road. Eventually the man set me down on the opposite pavement, and then, in the broadest Scottish accent, thought to ask me where I wanted to go. Getting my breath back with difficulty, I indicated the still rumbling engine and said, 'I want to get on that bus. I only want to go a short way.'

At that, this gigantic fellow began to roar with laughter. 'That's my lorry, love,' he spluttered. 'The next stop is Glasgow. When I saw you stick your arm out, I thought you needed a hand across the road.' He was kindness itself, and the joke had obviously made his day, but I couldn't help reflecting that, had he had smaller hands, I might have had an opportunity to speak before becoming airborne!

Although, in retrospect, this kind of experience has its funny side, it can be very disconcerting at the time. People who wish to give help are often reticent about doing so, because they simply don't know what to do. It is helpful if, as help is offered, it is accompanied by a light touch on the arm. In heavy traffic conditions, for instance, voices can merge into the general noise. I must say that the massive-hand-in-the-armpit experience was a unique one for me. More often one is held by the extreme tip of the elbow, and shunted, as it were, out into space. Most visually handicapped people prefer to take the the arm of the person who is guiding them, so that as the guide ascends and descends steps and kerbs fractionally before you, you can tell that your next step will be up or down. This is the way it works with a guide dog – the dog's front feet are ahead of its owner, and as it goes up and down kerbs the owner feels the angle of the rigid harness handle alter.

Another difficulty which sometimes arises is when a sighted person is showing someone who cannot see to a chair. More than once, after having been shunted around by the elbow method, and teetering through motions that closely resemble the steps of a dance, I have ended up sitting on the wrong side of a chair, with its back against one of my arms. The best way of avoiding this is simply to place a person's hand on top of the back of the chair. It doesn't take a moment, then, to ascertain which way round the chair is facing, and thus to make a more graceful landing and end up facing the right way. These very simple suggestions can help to avoid much embarrassment for all concerned.

Inevitably, though, there are times when you simply have to manage on your own. Going to the loo presented difficulties sometimes, especially if I was alone in a strange place. Usually, I would try to manage for as long as possible without going, but if it was absolutely necessary, I'd go with considerable misgivings, wondering if it was clean, trying not to touch the wall when feeling for the toilet roll or the chain. I hated old public loos where, when you were feeling around for the chain, you plunged your hand into a network of disgusting, dusty cobwebs.

Inevitably, I was also often asked how I felt about never having seen either of my two children. That first glimpse, when the new-born child is placed into its mother's arms, a living reality, must evoke an unsurpassable response in her heart. This, in normal circumstances, must be awakened through what the eye reports to the brain, and the brain transfers the message to wherever the home of love is in the human make-up. Never to have seen one's own baby must seem a denial of one of the most basic human joys and rights to those who have experienced its wonder. I answered quite truthfully that through my other senses I felt I had perceived every tiny detail of appearance and was aware of every mannerism. I had a complete and clear picture of both my sons in my mind, and did not feel the slightest tinge of regret.

I remember an incident a couple of years ago, when Ben was playing one of his interminable space games in the living-room. I was preparing the evening meal in the kitchen. A mixture of intuition and inspired guesswork told me that the settee had become the moon and that Ben was on a moon-walk, so I called to him to get off the settee. 'Oh Mum,' he said plaintively, 'I wish you weren't blind.' A dreadful pang went through me. Did this poor child feel some sort of deprivation because of my blindness? He went on, 'My friend's Mum doesn't know when we walk on her settee, and that's probably because she can see.'

Now the house was uncannily quiet – but not a quiet that caused me any pain. I knew that I had given all I could to our sons in those baby and toddler years. I do not mean by this that I had given them all I should: I was aware of my shortcomings as a mother, and therefore rejoiced in the confident hope that their days would now lead them to new horizons which I could only explore with them in imagination when they came home at teatime full of a new eagerness about a world for which I hoped I had equipped them adequately. Each morning, among all the little bits and pieces children carry in their school-bags, I tucked a little parcel of my love and prayers. They could not see it and probably never consciously found it, but I felt that these unseen offerings were the best I had.

During those full and busy days of school-teaching, and later the even busier days of motherhood, I had envied those who enjoyed a more leisurely way of life. I had envied, but would not have changed places, for at those times I had known that I was where I had to be, and wanted – even yearned – to be. Each part of the way, I was learning, had to be trodden in order for the full beauty of the next to be revealed.

It is odd that, being where we are, we often feel that we have failed. We look at others and wish we had what they have, were what they are, or what we think they are. When the children were tiny, on my rare shopping sprees to Derby, I would listen with envy to women in the restaurant who obviously met for lunch every week. Conversations overheard on buses revealed that women actually found time to read books, study psychology or even architecture. How I envied them their freedom, never stopping to think that maybe ten years, or even five years, earlier, they might have been in the position that I was in then.

Now my turn had come. We used our leisure, Martin and I, to meet friends for lunch and attend afternoon classes on literature, local stately homes and archaeology. How kind the other students in those classes were, often recording whole books for me when they were not available in Braille. I eagerly drank in every bit of knowledge I could get hold of, and allowed Jane Austen, Ibsen and Thomas Hardy to push 'Play School' and 'Magic Roundabout' gently out of the way. Public-speaking engagements came in thick and fast. Martin always stole the show whether our audience consisted of schoolchildren, Women's Institutes, or Rotary Clubs.

Everyone fell in love with my quiet companion, whose liquid brown eyes were far more eloquent than any words I could speak.

Gradually my batteries were recharged, and it seemed as though this gentle, pleasant time would go on for ever and ever. I felt that I had the best of several worlds – our pleasant home, the good company of friends, a certain amount of time on my hands to pursue my own interests, and the rough and tumble of the family coming in at teatime. I prided myself on always being there when the back door flew open, and the first word, 'Mum', was shouted at the top of the first voice, even if I was standing immediately inside that door. I glowed with pleasure if I happened to be upstairs when the second arrival was heralded with the question, 'Where's Mum?' They still needed me, and I needed to know that, even if it was not put into words.

It is perhaps a good thing that our lives, like the paths we tread, turn sudden, unexpected corners. Having become thoroughly used to, and at home with the old path, it is often not until much later that we realize the change of direction has been a blessing, even if somewhat heavily disguised at the time.

I was most certainly not expecting the slight accident Martin had one afternoon when we were all out walking on the moors. He fell and dislocated his shoulder, and we got him back to the car with great difficulty. It was not until we got home that we found the nasty gash on his chest. The vet made a marvellous job of dealing with his injuries, but Martin was almost twelve years old when that happened and his joints began to stiffen. He had worked well over the average estimated time, but a dog like him never seems to age. He still carried sticks half his own size again and scaled walls other dogs might turn away from.

About that time, too, I realized that his hearing was failing slightly, although he never missed out on supper duty. The opening of the fridge door, however quietly, still signifies that it is time for him to take up a sort of sentry-duty position by the kitchen worktop. It isn't that he's greedy, or really interested in the goings-on of the kitchen – you can tell by the expression of complete detachment on his face – but someone has to make sure these indolent humans don't drop pieces of cheese all over the kitchen floor and just leave them there. He learned years ago how remiss both Ian and I are in this respect.

As well as the stiffness and the deafness, I noticed that whereas at one time he would have woven our way in and out of a crowd, and had been known to startle people out of the way by applying his very cold, wet nose to the backs of their legs, he now quite often stood weighing up the situation and coming to a decision slowly.

Remembering how this faithful, unassuming and dependable friend of mine had been the channel for giving me back the freedom and independence I now valued so highly, I felt that if he was suffering any undue strain this state of affairs should not be prolonged. A visit from a guide dog trainer at Bolton confirmed my fears. Martin's age was beginning to tell on even his staunch spirit. We decided that I owed him as long and happy a retirement as possible. With Martin, I had long since been able to switch into what I called 'auto-dog', which meant that we seemed to read each other's minds and I needed to issue a bare minimum of commands. I knew that after ten years with this dog who, if I had let him, would not have been limited even by the sky, becoming accustomed to a successor was going to be tough.

It was not long before a suitable dog was ready.

One Friday in June 1985, Martin and I went into town

as usual for the weekly shop at the supermarket. We visited the greengrocer's, where Martin expects, and almost always gets, a small bunch of grapes. As usual, we called at a pub in the middle of town which serves coffee. There we met the usual crowd of Friday friends.

When we arrived home I slipped his harness off and rubbed his dear old domed head. He raised his face to mine and kissed my cheek. I think we both knew that never again would we walk where this trusty, dearest friend of friends and I had walked for so many years together. Never again would anyone say, 'Hello Martin. Have you brought your Mum shopping?' We both knew, I am sure, that that was the end of our partnership, but that the bond of friendship between us would remain strong and indestructible.

'Dear old friend,' I whispered in his long, silky ear. 'That funny domed head of yours has all the wisdom of Solomon inside it. You re-opened for me the highway to freedom, and all I can give you is my gratitude and love.' Were he not so wise and silent, and just a little bit more human, I'm sure he would have told me that that was all he would ask for. Many, many people offered Martin a home, and I am grateful to them, but without him our family would be incomplete. And who would supervise the supper?

CHAPTER 12

Victor

There were only five students on the training course this time and all of us were experienced guide dog owners. It seemed quiet in the spacious lounge, compared with the rumbustious crowd of ten years before. Val Woolrich had trained one of the dogs and had supervised an apprentice who had trained mine.

In the intervening ten years, Val and I had struck up a friendship, and had met socially on a number of occasions. This made not a scrap of difference to her attitude in class. I am not the best time-keeper in the world, although I always have watertight reasons for my lateness. These have not the slightest effect upon her, and one minute's delay finds her sitting at the wheel of the minibus surrounded by an atmosphere of uncrackable ice. Her attitude to my insistence on a daily shower, which interferes with a punctual start to breakfast, is less than sympathetic. The fact that I have failed to give the dog a hand-signal as well as a command is spotted by her from a distance of three miles and round several corners. For all that, she is firm and fair, and I trust her opinion on all matters concerning dogs implicitly.

On being told that this time my dog rejoiced in the name of Victor, I thought it was some sort of practical joke. No, that was the name I would have to go around enunciating loud and clear from now on. He is a cross-bred labrador and golden retriever, crossed with a golden retriever. It sounds complicated, but I reckon that makes him three-quarters golden retriever. For all that, he looks to the untrained eye just like a labrador, but taller. He is a very handsome dog, deep golden, with chocolate ears and tips, and a white chest and under-carriage. He has dark, kind eyes, and an inquisitive pinky-brown nose. I soon learned that he is what I call an extrovert-introvert. In other words, I believe that he is shy, sensitive and self-effacing, but doesn't want the world to recognize these basic characteristics in him. To cover up, he plays the part of a clown, standing on his head, bottom heavenward, lying gracelessly on his back, all four legs stretched stiffly in the air, or he sings a tuneless song, non-stop, and not made any more beautiful by the presence of somebody-or-other's shoe in his mouth.

The moment we met, I knew that here was a dog who would give me his all, provided I could give him constant encouragement and reassurance. My heart went out to him. I felt that during his short life he had given his heartful of love away three times – to his mother, his puppy-walker and his trainer – and each time had had to be passed along to the next link in the chain. How could I explain to him that I was the last link, that now there would be no more moves, and that at home there was a family longing to meet and love him?

We got off to a good start, but soon it looked as though things were going to go very seriously wrong. I had been under the weather for some weeks, with nothing in particular, but I was having difficulty sleeping. The strange bed and unfamiliar sounds at the training centre didn't do much to improve this. I was nervous about sleeping on the ground floor. A number of bedrooms were empty and I found the atmosphere rather eerie at night. I have always been uneasy with a new dog sleeping in my bedroom. The unfamiliar sounds disturb me, and I lie awake listening to them.

One night towards the end of the first week, I was

lying half-awake. Each time the dog moved in his sleep, his bed creaked and disturbed me. It was about three o'clock, that time when there is only the finest line between fantasy and reality. A low murmuring sound in the distance gradually increased in volume, as a gang of youths came nearer, obviously more than slightly drunk. I could not tell whether the sound belonged to the night or the day, but it came nearer and nearer. The side of the house on which I was sleeping faces the road, which is not far away at that point. In my half-awake state, I had forgotten this, and, leaping out of bed, grabbed the poor sleeping dog, slipped on his check chain and lead, and burst into my neighbour's room.

As it happened, we had trained together with our previous dogs ten years earlier, and we had remained good friends. Jill listened and summed up the situation immediately, but it was too late. By this time my imagination had run such a riot that I couldn't gather myself together. I understood the truth of the situation, but the fearful feeling inside refused to go. We sat chatting for a while. Just as I felt sufficiently composed to return to my room, Jill's dog began to make a noise we didn't recognize. Without stopping to think, or investigate, one of us pressed the emergency bell.

Within seconds Mrs Wood, the assistant matron, was with us. It was as well for us that she is an easy-going soul, with a lovely sense of humour. The sinister sounds Jill's dog was making were produced by nothing more formidable than a session of middle-of-the-night foot-washing.

Still strung up, I asked Mrs Wood if she would come back to my room, explaining that the dog's bed creaked and kept me awake. If we folded it away, he could sleep on the blanket. As the bed was taken down, it collapsed with a clatter that made us both jump, but Victor behaved

in the most unexpected way. He backed into a corner and
made the strangest noise – half-whimper, half-bark. I
was convinced by now that either he or I was going mad.
I jumped into bed and insisted that he should be taken
out of the room. Probably thinking me beyond hope, Mrs
Wood picked up poor Victor's lead and together they
marched out of the room.

What an utter fool I felt next morning when I awoke.
There was no Victor, and his bed stood, neatly folded,
against the wall. It really had happened then. How I
wished it had all been a dream. Now I really had blotted
my copy-book, and would probably be sent home
without a dog. At breakfast time I asked the kennel-maid
sitting beside me if she knew of Victor's whereabouts.
Giving nothing away, she informed me that he was
perfectly all right, and Miss Woolrich would sort out the
matter when she came in at 8.45.

My stomach was turning cartwheels that would have
graced any acrobatic performance. I had made an utter
fool of myself and had probably done untold harm to
poor Victor's psychological stability. After breakfast I sat
on my bed, utterly mortified. A light tap on the door
indicated that Miss Woolrich had come to 'sort things
out'. I explained as calmly as possible what had
happened.

There was not the slightest hint of criticism or blame in
her voice as she patiently explained that the time when a
dog is handed over from its trainer to its new owner can
be very traumatic for some of the more sensitive dogs.
This sometimes results in a dog behaving in a way that it
never has before. My fear in the night had obviously
communicated itself to Victor, and the noise made by the
bed collapsing was the final straw. The noises he had
then made were not aggressive, but were his way of
asking what on earth was going on. He would have been

completely bewildered by my unexpected reactions and fear.

'Have I done him any harm?' I asked, penitently. 'Well, you won't have done him much good, but I reckon he'll get over it,' I was reassured. 'So you're not sending me home without a dog?' I hardly dared put the question into words. 'Good heavens, no.' She sounded astonished. 'I am going to suggest that you have a hot milky drink, though, and go back to bed for the morning. You look terribly tired.' I had not expected that reaction but, doing as I was told, I slept soundly until lunchtime.

After lunch, Victor and I were reunited. He was obviously none the worse for the experience of the previous night. However, although he had shown no signs of wariness during his training, he always has a great deal to say about anything he meets for the first time. Guitars, trombones, tennis rackets, and a host of other fairly innocuous things have been the objects of much vocal abuse on his part. Victor has proved to be excellent at the work he was trained to do. But I learned that day that in order to get the best out of him, I had to give him plenty of reassurance: he needed me as much as I needed him. Isn't this the case, though, in any friendship? We each have our part to play. Without give and take, the relationship gets out of balance. Victor serves as a reminder that, however well a dog may be treated, its training does not make it into a robot or a machine.

That night we all went out to a local pub. I think everyone was determined that if we couldn't beat them, we'd join them. By the time we had finished the first round, everyone was able to joke about the previous night's walkabout. Val Woolrich described how she had arrived at work that morning to find Anne, who had trained Victor, and Mark, an apprentice trainer, standing together with the bleakest expressions on their faces. She couldn't help but know that something had gone drastically wrong, and framed her opening question accordingly.

'Victor spent the night with one of the kennel staff,' she was told. 'Mrs T. wouldn't have him in her room. She was certain he was going to attack her. Isn't it awful? Whatever will happen?' They were staggered by Val's calm reception of these tidings. 'Oh, is that all? She threw a wobbler during the first week when she trained with Martin. This can be a stressful time for some people. Now it's out of her system. Don't worry, it's the way she functions.' How perceptive, and how factually correct. With that sorted out, we could get down to the serious business of the training course.

Transferring one's trust from a previous dog to a new one is not automatic, and often not easy. Although we are strongly urged by the trainers not to do so, it is almost impossible not to make comparisons between the two. The new dog has to be taught to walk in straight lines, except where obstacles make this impossible, and to turn left, right, or back, on command. He stops at kerbs, refusing to cross until the road is clear. Flights of steps are clearly indicated by the dog sitting down at the top or bottom of them. In every respect, the dog is equipped to lead a blind person safely through the many conditions encountered in the course of daily living. What no instructor can teach a dog is the individual rapport that will develop between it and the owner with whom it will spend the major part of its working life. Martin and I seemed to know each other's mind. Building the relationship is not very different from developing a human friendship – it requires time, patience, and a certain amount of self-sacrifice. The resulting reward makes it more than worthwhile giving all three.

* * *

Two or three days before we were due to go home, Jenny, who had been Victor's puppy-walker, arrived to collect her current puppy from the training centre, where he had been kennelled while she was away on holiday. I felt privileged to meet the person who had devoted hours of love and patience to the dog who was now to become my eyes.

From the age of six weeks, until they are about a year old, the puppies live with a family where, in every respect, they are treated as family pets. They are taught to be obedient and sociable, learning to recognize basic commands, such as 'Sit', 'Down' and 'Stay'. They are taught to walk on an ordinary leash, but slightly in front of the handler, not to heel as a puppy would normally walk. Gradually the young guide-dog-to-be is introduced to the kind of conditions he is likely to come across if he makes the grade. He is taken into shops and restaurants, railway stations and libraries, and taught to curl up under the seat on buses. He is introduced to as many people as possible, and actively discouraged from asking for or accepting tit-bits. Each month the pup is visited and walked by the puppy-walking supervisor, who assesses his progress and gives advice where needed. Just when the pup has learned all about law and order, and has ceased to be hard work, when puddle days and chewing days are at an end, or almost, along comes the supervisor to take him back to the centre to begin his special training for the work of guiding.

Is it just a coincidence that a fluffy little bundle tumbles out of the back of the car and looks appealingly at the bereft angel who does a job that few would envy? Yet not many of these invaluable people stop after the first pup has been parted with. But oh, the pride and joy they feel, around a year later, on receiving a photograph of the fully trained dog, looking resplendent in a white harness and gazing lovingly at a brand-new blind owner. This must do much to offset the grief felt at parting after the first essential part of the dog's training has been accomplished.

Victor had been Jenny's third puppy. She had been struck by his sensitivity, all wrapped up in a packing of boisterousness. Her heart had gone out to the lost look in the baby brown eyes. It had not taken her long to realize that, as long as he received masses of encouragement, there was nothing that this dog would not do. She never pushed or hurried him, and found that in this way she could encourage him to have a go at almost anything.

Jenny told me of how she had taken Victor to a lake on the moors near her home. Her previous pups had loved water and she was surprised when it became obvious that the sight of the lake terrified Victor. At first his temporary Mum just splashed her hand at the edge, chatting to the puppy to help him feel at ease. The next time she dropped twigs into the water, near enough to the edge for him to be able to fish them out with a paw. This continued for several visits, the sticks being thrown a little further out each time. Then one day, Victor suddenly leapt into the lake without realizing what he was doing and instantly showed himself to be an extremely strong swimmer.

I remember well the first Christmas after I had him. Ian was in bed with flu, and the rest of us went with some friends for a walk by the river near our home. The snow was deep and frozen solid. It was very cold. All of a sudden, a splash told me what I would rather not have known. That great golden nut had jumped into the freezing water. When he came out, the water on his coat instantly turned to hundreds of tiny icicles.

Jenny writes poems about her pups, and on Valentine's Day, not long after he had left her, Victor received a Valentine card from her. Inside was a very moving poem she had written to him. After that he was known at the centre as Victor Valentine. I was moved almost to tears when Jenny produced from her bag two shields and three certificates which had been awarded to Victor during his year with her. She always takes her guide dog pups along to obedience training night with her own pet dog, and Vic had managed to gain some first and second places. We are always astonished by this, as it took me a whole year to teach him to give a paw. The boys love to tease him about it.

The work that Jenny and all puppy-walkers do is messy and often frustrating, but absolutely invaluable to the Association. Warm-hearted, generous Jenny gave me many insights into Victor's character by recounting stories of his baby months, and I am sure that others would say the same of those who puppy-walked their dogs. Vic has just received his fifth birthday card from her.

When we arrived home, I think my friends had expected the new dog to be a younger replica of Martin. I think that is what I had subconsciously imagined, too. Imagine their utter amazement when they were greeted by a flying mass of legs, head and tail that never stopped talking and used unrepeatable language if they happened to be carrying anything he didn't like the look of – ladders, buckets, etc. When Victor is particularly pleased to see somebody he grabs a wrist and leads him or her into the house. For those who were used to Martin's dignified, rather autocratic way, this could be open to misinterpretation. I went to great lengths to convince callers – and, perhaps, myself – that all this noise and wrist-grabbing were expressions of friendship.

Among my treasures I had placed the shields Victor had been awarded, and the certificate which spoke of his

tenacity by certifying that at the age of eleven months he
had, with Jenny's husband Eric, walked thirty-six miles
in ten-and-a-half hours. And then there were all those
poems written by one who had loved him, admired his
beauty, encouraged him, and had faith in him. If Victor
did not reach his full potential and become all that Martin
had been as a guide, it must not be because I had denied
him that same degree of love and trust and faith. Ours
was a partnership and I must make sure that my side of it
was sound and firm and reliable, too.

We were thrown in at the deep end. My diary was full
of speaking engagements, and more and more I was
being asked to open summer, autumn, spring and
Christmas fairs, carnivals, and other functions where the
proceeds were being donated to the work of the Guide
Dogs for the Blind Association. Solemn old Martin had
walked at my side, regal and wise, looking the part in
every respect, from the tip of his wet black nose to the tip
of his feathery cream tail. Now I was called upon to
assume an air of calm dignity, while hissing gentle words
of admonition under my breath, unobserved I hoped,
and keeping a restraining hand upon this frisking,
dancing two-year-old, inquisitive pink nose in the air
sniffing out mischief, with mouth open ready to assist
with my speech. He bore little resemblance in those early
days to everyone's idea of what a guide dog should be,
but he certainly endeared himself to all who met him. It
was not long before our local shopkeepers, traffic
wardens and lollipop ladies had given their hearts to
Victor, in much the same way as they had to Martin.

Now, a few years on, there has been little change in the
exuberant mouth-and-tail greeting, the contents of the
shoe-cupboard still litter the floor in a trail from stairs to
basement, my talks are often accompanied or punctuated
by a low whining; but every day I walk out in familiar and

unfamiliar places, fully confident that the golden friend with chocolate ears that still skips by my side, will not let me down and we shall arrive safely home when our work is done.

Martin eyed the newcomer with quiet disdain. He did not condescend to communicate with him, except that, if we were walking in the countryside and Victor had the effrontery to creep up from behind and relieve him of one of the three or four sticks he always carries, from the corner of Martin's mouth issued language I had never heard him use before. Victor, on the other hand, adores Martin and looks for him around the house on the days when he goes visiting one of his many friends. On a number of occasions during the first few months, Martin pushed his head through the harness when I held it out. Only the fact that the strap, set for Victor's girth, was too tight to accommodate Martin's more ample proportions, denied him a trip out with me to visit his old haunts. But he soon settled contentedly to 'guard the house' when he saw me gathering my 'going out' things together, knowing that sooner or later a walk in the fields would give him the exercise and fun he so enjoys.

CHAPTER 13

Back in Harness

At about this time, several of my friends who are teachers or nurses began to return to work part-time, or even full-time. Our children were becoming less dependent, and in these professions there was always plenty of temporary part-time work to be had. I envied them their independence. They jumped into their cars after their children had gone to school and drove off into a world in which I had no part.

During the last dozen or so years, these friends and I had shared our joys and heartaches and knew each other almost as well as we knew ourselves. Now they were driving off into what seemed to me, from my position at the kitchen sink, a world of excitement and glamour. In my mind's eye, I saw them as giants of womanhood. I listened wistfully as their cars roared further and further away, and the note of the engine became a deep, throbbing beat, and then finally a silence which I could reach out and touch. And then my heart would throb, too, and throbbed on, until it became a deep, silent ache.

Why did I ache and grieve so much? The captive lion lifts his head at sunset and roars plaintively for the freedom of his native land, the place where he should be. I would have laughed if, fourteen years before, anyone had told me that one day I would yearn again for the buzz and chatter and activity of a classroom full of children. I would not have believed the smell of pencils and books and half-eaten sweets stowed away in warm pockets would evoke in me such nostalgic memories that just thinking of them set me on fire with a longing to be back

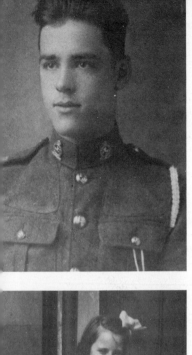

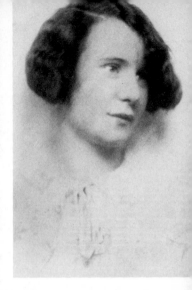

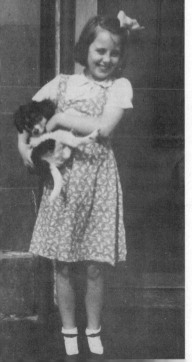

Above: My father and mother before they were married.

Left: There was always a pet dog in my parents' home, and I loved each of them dearly, thinking of them as friends and playmates. I had very little sight left by this time.

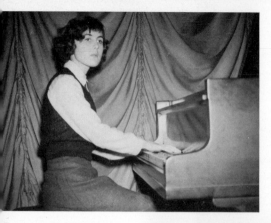

Left: I was very nervous indeed as I waited to play the piano before an invited audience who had come to see a film, *Pathway into Light*, which had been made to commemorate the centenary of Louis Braille.

Right: Jean Metcalfe was as warm in person as was the voice I had heard so often on the radio, introducing the programme 'Forces' Favourites'. As I stood beside her on the stage in the small Oxford Street cinema, I realized that I was not dreaming as the familiar voice announced that I was now going to play Schumann's Romance in F sharp major.

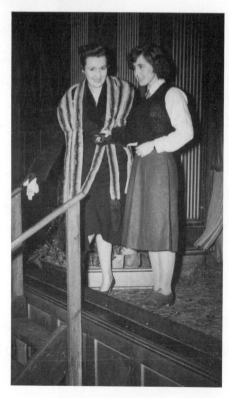

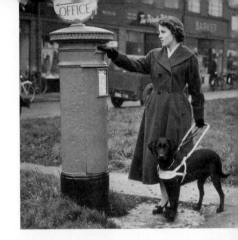

Right: 'Find the post box' was one of the many instructions Neana learned to recognize and obey.

Below: Neana kept a watchful eye upon my pupils as I read to them from a textbook which, of course, was in Braille.

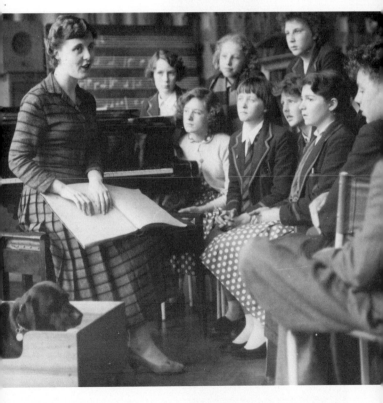

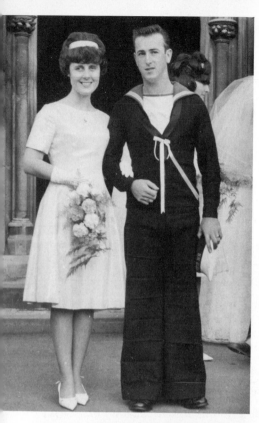

Left: My brother Nick was married during his nine years' naval service.

Below: Ian and I were married at St Peter's Church, Belper, in the lovely month of April 1971. It was Easter Monday. Everything in nature spoke of new life.

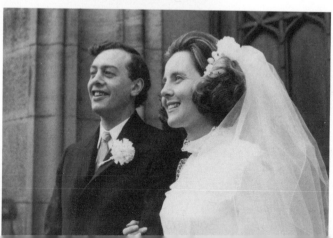

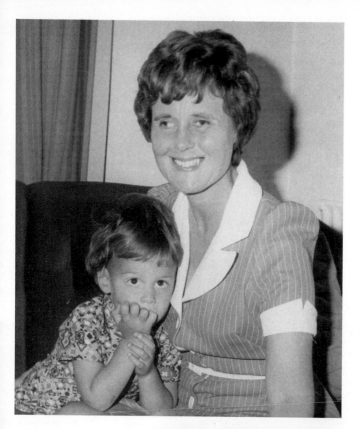

Above: Adam was always eager for a story.

Derby Evening Telegraph

Right: I spent several lovely holidays with my former college friend Pam and her husband David, at their home in Salisbury. Dana, of course, was included in the invitation.

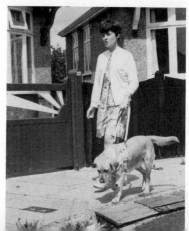

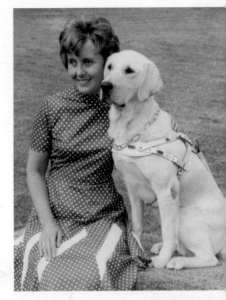

Right: Martin, the gentle giant, sat beside me on our last day at the Bolton guide dog training centre. He was about to begin his ten years of service as my faithful friend and trusty guide.

Below: No words could adequately express the depth of emotion I felt the first few times I saw my children. This photo shows Ben visiting me in hospital.

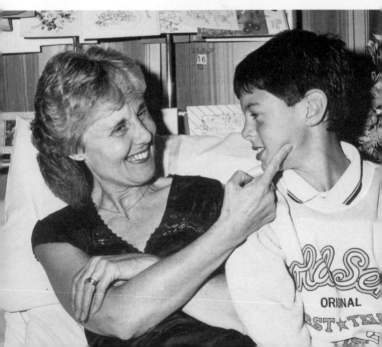

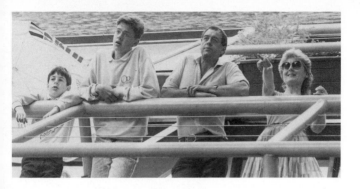

Above: It was a perfect summer day when, at the end of August 1987, a local newspaper invited my family and me to spend a day visiting some of the beautiful places in Derbyshire which I had long loved, but never seen. As we stood on the balcony of the restaurant at Matlock's cable car station, I was thrilled by the valley's depth and the grandeur of the hills beyond. *Trader Group of Newspapers*

Below: The money raised by Butterley Police Headquarters will pay for the rearing and basic training of the puppies Bonnie and Clyde (in the framed photograph). With Ian and me are Ivan Bamford (left) and Inspector Brian Cain with Mrs Rebecca Smith (Mish) second from left.

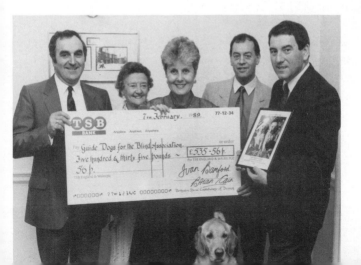

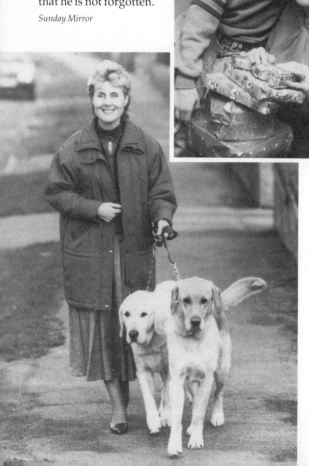

Right: Christmas 1987 was a strange mixture of thrilling new experiences, bright colours and simple homely pleasures.
Sunday Mirror

Below: Victor always enjoys an off-duty run, and Martin makes sure that he is not forgotten.
Sunday Mirror

there in the middle of it all. I remembered, as I stood by the washing machine, turning socks the right way out and scrubbing the shirt collars, that feeling of achievement when a point you have been trying to get over suddenly goes home, and you feel three dozen pairs of eyes gaze at you as understanding dawns. The memories would crowd in, and the teacher inside went on knock, knock, knocking to be set free.

Friends and family encouraged me to apply to become a supply teacher, but I knew that I had completely lost my nerve. The whole system of education had changed since I had left the classroom. Large comprehensive schools had replaced the smaller secondary moderns and grammar schools. I had no experience of teaching mixed-ability classes. I did not any longer recognize the names of the subjects – even they had all changed. The age of technology had hit the classroom in a big way, and it all seemed beyond my understanding. Apart from all this, there were such dreadful stories about today's young people, the lack of discipline and decline in standards. It all sounded terrifying.

I was talking this over with a teacher one day, and she said she felt I would find it very difficult to cope with today's climate in the classroom. At one time that would have been all I needed to spark off the fight to prove to myself and to the world in general that I would not let a handicap stand in the way of something I was determined to do. The fight had gone, though. For the very first time in my life, I began to think of myself as a handicapped person and, worse, that the handicap made me inferior to others. I did not discuss this despair even with those nearest to me. Defeated I might be, but I didn't want anyone to know of the humiliation that defeat caused me.

Victor and I continued with the round of talks and

public functions. What a paradox that at this time it was always being remarked that I was poised, confident and calm. No one could see the little bird with the broken wing that fluttered feebly inside, unable to rise and soar into the beckoning skies. I could hear, as though it were a thousand miles away, the confident, cheerful voice that had listeners weeping and laughing in turns as the tale was told, but only my heart heard the little bird with the broken wing, sobbing softly inside.

To make matters worse, I despised this wretched, pathetic individual who, for the first time, minded, really minded, being blind.

Sitting in a café one filthy wet morning, I heard the women in the kitchen laughing and joking. They have an identity, I thought. They work at the café. I can teach, but no one would want me, because I am blind. Why had God dangled the world in front of me, like a great Technicolor ball, only to take it away again? Now it's dark here, and I'm afraid.

Of course, I was not so downcast all the time. Through my dogs and public speaking, I was happy to be meeting some of the many hundreds of people, of all ages and from all walks of life, who devote hours of time and energy to helping those less fortunate than themselves. Nor was there any time for regret and self-pity when the door burst open towards the end of each afternoon and the boys exploded through the doorway, scattering shoes and football gear, attacking the biscuit tin as though tomorrow would be the first day of a famine, and in general causing the sort of chaos that a mother views with horror and affection. 'Where's Mum?' reminded me that they needed me, even if the rest of the world didn't seem to.

'What an incredible waste of all that education,' I grumbled, as I trudged wearily up the stairs, arms full of newly ironed washing, precariously balanced, and held together at the top by the tip of my nose. 'I little thought,' I muttered on, voice muffled by the neatly folded garments coming between my protestations and the outer world, 'that I'd end up as nothing more than a washerwoman.' The rather loud pop music issuing from my elder son's room indicated that he had heard this speech, or variations of it, sufficiently often to be completely unimpressed.

It was a beautiful summer morning, and when the boys had at last got off to school, and the house had settled into the sort of comfortable quiet that breathes through it when I'm here with the dogs, my hand touched the basket of unironed clothes on the kitchen table. They seemed to grin up at me with malicious humour. 'Ha, ha. Here we are, still waiting to be ironed,' they seemed to say. I'm sure the bottom of that pile doesn't really exist. This was a gruesome assortment – all shirts and frilly blouses. I needed a cup of coffee before I tackled that lot.

Something deep down in my subconscious always recommends a cup of coffee as soon as the door shuts behind those two sons of mine. Retrieving football boots that Vic has carried off, rescuing homework that has somehow found its way into the bin, finding a plastic carrier bag for the swimming gear and generally keeping everyone's time-schedule going – as well as making sure someone feeds the guinea-pig – leaves me feeling slightly bedraggled. I owed myself the luxury of a cup of coffee.

Sitting down to drink it, I was startled by the ringing of the phone. I recognized the voice of Mary Mason, a former colleague, now acting head of our old school. I assumed she was going to ask me to talk to the children at assembly.

'Judy,' I heard her saying, 'I'm absolutely desperate. I

can't get hold of any supply teachers, and I need someone for music. Would you come in for the day?'

'Me? I'm not even dressed. I'd be terrified. I must be horribly out of date and – well, do you think I could manage?'

The calm voice assured me that I'd be fine, and that I could have the old music-room. I promised to get there as soon as possible. I took particular care over my dress and make-up, shoved a couple of cassettes in my bag, sorted out a friend to give Martin a run, and Vic and I set off.

Sitting on the bus that day in July 1986, the warm sun streaming through the window and caressing my cheek with reassuring friendliness, I wanted to shout at the top of my voice, 'I am here because somebody needs me today. I am here because someone has faith in me. She said she was desperate, and thought of me.'

Heavens! That struck a familiar note somewhere. Thirty years before, that same word 'desperate' in Miss Baxter's letter from Rugby had broken through the dark glass of my gloom and let the sunbeams in, giving me a chance to dance along life's path. Could this really be happening to me, or was I just day-dreaming beside the basket of ironing, trying to convince myself that I, like my friends in their cars, could roar off into the magical world of work?

The bus stopped with a jolt. 'We're there, duck,' the driver called back to me. He was a former pupil of mine, and 'duck' is a form of endearment in these parts. 'Are you going to give them a talk?' he asked.

'No, they need me to do a day's teaching,' I said loudly and, I hoped, with a note that would convey the importance of the occasion in my voice.

As Victor and I walked along the once so familiar drive, the messages my brain was endeavouring to send to my feet just didn't seem to reach their destination. This must be how men felt when they went moon-walking. My mind went back many years, to a conference house in which I had stayed. It was mid-winter, and exceedingly cold. I had needed to go to the bathroom in the night. My slippers wouldn't fit over the bedsocks I was wearing against the Arctic conditions, and the corridor was carpeted with coconut matting, to which the big, woolly socks stuck stubbornly as I tried to lift my feet. Each step was a real labour, and the trip took so long that someone came after me, thinking I had got locked in. Now, with my heart beating at what seemed twice its normal rate, I struggled with my feet, each feeling as though it weighed a ton. There were no children around. That would give me a chance to practise walking along the corridor looking like a teacher, not like a frightened rabbit that had no right to be there.

I must have looked pretty scared, because the moment I timidly put my head round the staffroom door, I was invited to sit down and a cup of coffee was thrust into my trembling hand. The staff came in for break. A former colleague spotted me, and beamed good-humouredly. 'Well, well, have they had to bring you out of cold storage?' he asked. Then Victor, obviously feeling it was about time someone noticed him, stood on his head and sang a short, fairly tuneless song in his best baritone voice. The ice was immediately broken; I relaxed and gathered together my bags and books, hoping I looked more impressive than I felt.

A senior member of staff accompanied me to the music-room. Nothing had changed there. The piano, the record player, the filing cabinet, were all exactly where they had been fourteen years before. The same sounds drifted along from the gym, and just outside children were practising for sports day. 'Nothing's changed,' I remarked to my kind helper. He felt, however, that one or two pieces of advice would not go amiss. 'You'll find the kids a lot noisier now,' he told me, 'and things aren't as formal these days, although we do try to keep up standards here.'

Then the class was there, running, sliding, shuffling to their places. I wondered if I should apologize that they wouldn't have a 'proper' teacher today. Just as I was debating the matter with myself, I heard the old, familiar sound of someone slinging his school-bag across the room. Before I had time to stop her, the one-time confident, rather formidable disciplinarian in me had leapt out and was dealing with the unsuspecting child in no uncertain terms. That was it. Our relationship was established. We all knew exactly where we were and, old-fashioned or not, a good working relationship was established.

As the class listened to the record of 'Tubby the Tuba' and dutifully turned in their books to the picture of each instrument when it was mentioned, I became aware of a familiar sound. I had heard it often at home. Someone was playing with something. Ben had a toy that made that sound when he tried to hide it under the dinner table.

Making a wild and shamefully sexist guess, I said quietly, 'Would the young man who finds his toy car more interesting than the music bring it here, please.' The 'young man', for the guess had been an inspired one, reluctantly handed over the car, and then, for good measure, delved into his pocket, and produced two more. As the class left the room, I heard him muttering to his friend, 'I thought she was supposed to be blind.'

Before the next lesson, a considerate member of staff reminded Mary that there were a couple of notorious miscreants in the class I would be teaching and offered to have them herself. 'Don't worry,' he was told, 'Judy will manage them.'

Such faith! What's more, such faith in me. She could not have known what that declaration of confidence did for me. She was speaking of the 'me' she had known, not of the 'me' I thought I had become. In that moment, I felt myself grow inches taller, self-respect and a new confidence flooded in. The realization that my friend and former colleague had had enough faith in my abilities to call upon me at very short notice and trust me to cope with classes, out of practice as I was, and was now quite sure that I would cope, unaided, with a potentially difficult group, filled me with renewed hope.

We had fun, the children and I, for the rest of that day. There is a sort of laughter-making banter that belongs to a happy classroom. To outsiders I suppose it would all sound rather silly, but teachers and their pupils spend many hours of their lives together, and a wise teacher quickly learns that laughter and learning can walk hand in hand.

When I got home, I was so exhilarated by the unexpected events of the day that I laughed triumphantly in the glum face of the ironing basket. The creased garments were still sulking away there on the kitchen table, but with a vigour I had not felt for months I soon smoothed them into a crisp, neat pile and then recounted all that had happened to the family, certain that they would be really impressed that, for one whole day, their Mum had been a real working woman.

Until the end of term, my services were required a number of times. My heart warmed as I walked along the corridor and heard children exclaim, 'Oh good, Mrs Taylor and Victor are here.' I soon learned that all the smart new names for the subjects taught and the strange titles denoting a teacher's position in the school are little more than a sign of the age of technology in which we live. There is certainly no need to be intimidated by them. Children are still children and, I soon realized, still respond to a teacher who is firm and fair.

My boys' relationships with each of the dogs are very different. When Martin sits up, looking wise and regal, and obviously taking it as a very personal insult that he is not included when the sandwich plate is offered to each of us in turn, I can hear a note almost of embarrassment in their voices as they instruct him to 'Lie down'. It is almost as if they were asking Grandad if he had washed his hands before coming to the table.

Victor, in contrast, has been nominated the family comedian, and accepts his role more than happily. That evening of my first day supply teaching I heard the friendly banter in the living room: 'How do you like being a schoolboy, Vic? Have they managed to teach you anything yet? Martin never went to school, but Martin didn't need to.' No, I reflected in the kitchen, it does seem as though Martin was born knowing most things. Victor, basking in the attention he so much enjoys, demonstrated his aptitude for learning by rushing off and bringing yet another shoe to add to those already scattered through most of the house.

I hope that I have not made Martin sound too good to be true. That would be unfair to him. For one thing, he has a delightful sense of humour – a quality which often seems to be lacking in out-and-out goodie-goods. For another, he does have one particular failing, which has often caused me considerable embarrassment. Although in every other respect he is a highly intelligent dog, I have come to the conclusion that there is a loose connection somewhere between his brain and his appetite – the two just don't seem ever to communicate.

A model of perfection, and, I might say, a perfect gentleman whenever he went with me to church, Martin would even stand for the Creed and bow his head respectfully for the blessing. When he accompanied me to church for a choral wedding, I handed him over to the person doing duty as verger, by whose side he would obediently stay until I returned to the vestry. He would not even give any sign of recognizing me until the vestry door was closed, and then he would leap all over me, pleased to be reunited. During the intervening half-hour, though, he could be counted on to sit majestically at his post and beam a welcome to all the guests. Many a nervous bride has been reassured by his charming smile.

It was because of his blameless record there that, one Sunday evening, I had no qualms about urging him 'Forward' to the communion rail, where small, chatting children are regularly smiled upon and blessed. At my command, he sat, and I knelt in the space to which he had guided me.

Imagine the dilemma in which I found myself when, just as the communion bread was being placed in my upturned palm, I heard a loud 'sniff, sniff, sniff' beside my left ear, and felt the bulk of furry, canine shoulders forcing their way between myself and the next communicant. I knew that if I didn't act with haste, the plate would be wiped clean, so, trying to preserve a reverent expression, I shoved my left elbow under his chin and managed to avert an ecclesiastical crisis. I really thought no one had noticed, but on the way out of church, the Vicar solemnly shook me by the hand and remarked, 'We shall have to have that fellow confirmed.'

On another occasion, we were queuing at the checkout of our local supermarket. I was thinking mildly uncharitable thoughts about the small children who were racing around apparently unobserved by their preoccupied mothers. Martin was sitting, a model of perfection, by my side. Suddenly, I felt his head go down for one brief moment, but I didn't attach any importance to it. After a longish wait I paid for my goods, packed them in

my bag, and marched to the main doors outside which a
large crowd waited for the bus.

'Oh, Mrs Taylor,' someone in the crowd said, a note of
horror in her voice. 'Martin's got a paper bag in his
mouth.' She named a local baker's shop, where the
confectionery is by no means cheap.

Conscious that more than a few pairs of eyes were
watching us – some amused, others amazed – I knew that
I must be seen to be taking action against this lovable
miscreant. And I knew that the crowd would be on his
side! I rather wished that the store manager would come
and deal with this shoplifter. He would be more able to
make a professional job of 'apprehending him on the
pavement outside the premises'.

Trying to pretend I couldn't hear the 'Ooohs' and 'Ahs'
and 'Look at his sweet little face' remarks that were being
exchanged, I put on a very severe expression, and in
what I considered my best 'playground' voice, I
demanded of Martin, 'What have you got there, my boy?'

Bending down, I relieved him of the bag, which was
dangling at a rakish angle from the corner of his mouth,
and plunged my hand into it. My fingers sank into a
sticky, gooey mass of cream and jam, and through it all
identified the more solid part of a doughnut. As I
withdrew my hand, the piece of mangled confectionery
came out with it, firmly impaled upon my fingers.

It was a very hot summer's day, and within moments
the cream started to drip, completely out of control. The
next moment, I nearly joined the 'out of control' part of it.
A spiteful buzzing, which heralds the approach of a wasp
and which my ears pick up from yards away, caused me
to forget all about the severity and dignity I had
mustered. I am very allergic to wasp stings, and find it
impossible even to pretend to be calm when they are
anywhere around.

'What shall I do with it?' I appealed to the crowd, holding up the rapidly melting mass.

'Give it 'im, duck,' was the first piece of advice I received and, putting the disapproval of every guide dog trainer I had ever known temporarily out of my mind, I thrust the disgusting object into Martin's already open mouth. Three months later, a lady came up to me in the street and told me that it was her shopping bag that Martin had raided that day, and as she had sat eating her cakeless lunch, she had reflected that there was no one else she would rather have shared it with.

To be fair, there was one occasion when good nature and perfect training prevailed over basic, brutish instinct, and we were truly impressed.

I was hanging washing on the line, and Martin was sniffing around the garden. Ian had gone into town, but I knew he wouldn't be too long. A number of birds had already flown into the glass of our conservatory and had either been killed or quite badly stunned, so I knew exactly what had happened when I heard a loud thud and then something drop just inside the back gate.

Martin ran over to investigate, and immediately I gave the command 'Sit, and stay', which he obeyed. Afraid that Ian would open the gate and damage the bird further, if indeed it were still alive, I stood guard and Martin sat quite still beside me.

Eventually, when Ian arrived, I warned him about the bird; as he looked over the top of the gate, the poor creature started to flutter into life and after a moment or two spread its wings and prepared to fly off. As it rose into the air, Martin, without warning, leapt several feet from the ground and caught it in his mouth. 'Leave it,' Ian yelled. Rather to the amazement of both of us, Martin opened his mouth, releasing his captive. It flew off, apparently none the worse for the double adventure.

CHAPTER 14

Prayer Power

Over the years I have come to know well a number of the social workers for the visually handicapped that have visited me in the course of their duties. Each has brought with her her own particular gifts, and each has made her own special mark upon my life. In one way and another, I am indebted to every one of them. I do not believe our lives ever cross the path of another without leaving something of their individual hues and tints behind. We are rather like the threads that make the warp and weft of a great cloth woven by an unseen craftsman. The threads, each with their individual colours and textures, are mingled and intertwined. Each thread lends something of itself to those around it, and myriads of new tones and tints emerge to delight the craftsman's eye.

One day during that summer of 1986, in the school holidays, Wendy, the social worker for this area arrived for what I thought was to be a routine call. I always enjoy her visits. She shares my love of pretty clothes, and we seem to have similar tastes in perfume. I value the advice she has given me on colour, particularly with regard to make-up.

For most women – and men, for that matter – their awareness of what is happening in the world of fashion is through what they see on television and in magazines and shop-windows. For blind women, to whom these sources of information are not available in the same way, it would be easy to wear clothes that look dowdy and old-fashioned. I have always been keenly interested in fashion – it has almost become a hobby. So when Wendy told me that she had arranged for a beauty and colour analyst to run a beauty workshop the following week for those of her clients who would be interested, I needed no second invitation. The workshop was a tremendous success. I was amazed at how adventurous I became as a result of it, even daring to blend together three shades of eye-shadow, a thing I would never have thought possible.

I learnt that Lea, our teacher, trained others to become beauty and colour analysts, and asked if I could attend the sessions held at her home on Monday evenings. It seems rather a daft idea, now I think about it, but at the time I was eager to learn all I could about the subject. Every Monday evening I turned up dutifully, and more often than not found myself in the model's chair. The others were always friendly, and never excluded me from the discussions, but I am sure that secretly they must have found the situation quite incongruous. For my own part, I did actually enjoy the talks and demonstrations, and did not feel I was wasting my time.

One evening several of the women said that they would not be able to attend the following Monday, as they were going to a four-night conference on 'Healing in the Church Today' at a church in Derby. It appeared that several teams from an American church which was renowned for its powerful healing ministry were visiting churches all over England, and one of the teams was coming to Derby.

It surprised me to find that about half the class was going to the conference, and I was rather disappointed that I had known nothing about it. Although I myself knew little about healing, I did know several people who believed that they had been healed through the prayers of their friends, and I had even heard talks by practising doctors who believed that prayer and medicine should go hand in hand. The subject fascinated me, and I wanted to know more about it.

I certainly had no thought of asking for healing for myself just then. I had a feeling that, if God did want to use my life in any way, it would not actually matter too much whether I was blind or not. In any case, as I have said before, my handicap never seemed a great disaster to me. It had certainly not interfered with my career, and my family were apparently not in the least put out by it.

All the same, I really did wish I had been able to go to the conference. Therefore, when Lea arrived at our house next evening and said that she would be going herself and would get a ticket for me, if I wished, I was astonished and delighted.

As I sat in the large, crowded church the following Friday evening, my mind was full of thoughts of a very close friend who had recently had a seriously handicapped baby. I knew that she was often sad and perplexed, and I wanted to know how best I could help her. I hoped that I might hear some of the answers at the conference.

Towards the end of the second evening, two ladies, strangers to me, came at separate times and told me that they were certain I would be healed. I thanked them, but would have liked to have told them not to get concerned on my behalf, as I had not come with any thought of asking for healing for myself.

On Sunday and Monday nights, towards the end of the service, a number of people gathered round me and prayed that my sight would be restored. The air was full of something indescribably beautiful – hope, and trust, and love. There was a feeling that God was very near.

A member of the American team then joined our group, a man full of good humour and fun. (It is sad that those of us who believe that God created the world sometimes seem to have forgotten that he must therefore have created laughter. What a pity we all too often hear prayers offered up in dreary, agonized voices.) After what seemed to me like hours, Jesse Lee – the big, friendly American – told us that he was quite certain that our prayers would be answered, but he was just as certain that members of our own church were to do the praying.

It all seemed very wonderful at the time, but in the cold light of the next day, I must admit that I began to get cold feet about the whole thing. Indeed, I felt rather embarrassed about it all. It was not that I did not have complete faith that God can do all things, but now, with the sink full of dirty dishes and the boys' shoes in a heap by the back door, just where they'd kicked them off as usual, now that everything was back to mundane everydayishness, I couldn't understand why everyone was so keen for me to have something I could manage perfectly well without. All the same, I reflected, washing up a tea-bag and putting the spoon into the rubbish bin, all the same, how privileged I was to have friends with such faith on my behalf that they had gone on knocking at the gates of heaven for years, and were certainly not going to let it go now.

It was not long before life had settled back into the usual routine. It was almost Christmas, and there were so many other things to think of that I, for one, felt I was far too busy to fit an extra meeting into the week. Anyway, I was still feeling somewhat embarrassed about the whole thing, although I still had to admit that it had been a very real experience at the time.

The supply teaching at Belper School seemed to have dried up, so I was absolutely delighted when a senior teacher at St Benedict's, a Catholic comprehensive school about seven miles away, rang and asked if I would like to do some supply teaching there. Apparently, a mutual friend had mentioned my name. Thereafter, I went in on the bus every Friday.

Victor loves going to school and always makes numerous friends, in both the staffroom and the class-room. At Belper School, a number of the pupils knew me through their parents, many of whom had been my pupils in the past, and once we had met and I had explained the circumstances to the class, I encountered few problems with which any sighted teacher would not have been faced. I started by telling the children that anyone who knew the answer to a question that I might ask should say my name, for the more conventional hand waving in the air was likely to be left there until its owner's circulation had quite stopped. I always insisted, for the sake of my own neck's wellbeing, that school-bags should be tucked right away under chairs. Very often, at first, the children were so fascinated by the fact that I could correctly identify fidgeting noises without actually being able to see them that they were tempted to play little games of 'spot the noise' with me. However, this game soon lost its charm for them when they discovered that, because I had their academic progress so much at heart, the time these games took to play would have to be made up for in the official breaks. It was not long before, just as in the old days, a hand would be slipped through my arm in a crowded corridor, and a youngster would volunteer to accompany me to the staffroom.

The other noteworthy event of January 1987 was that one of my friends, Sally, thought it high time the prayer group got under way and called a meeting for all who were interested. Thereafter, half-a-dozen to a dozen people, men and women, met every Monday evening in the home of one or other of the members. I was astonished by the faith of all those who came. I have to admit that my own faith, at times, by no means matched theirs.

After all, I had seen nothing but light in one eye, and the other eye had been completely blind, for many years. Specialists, over that time, had reluctantly said that they could do nothing to help me. I had considerable disorders of the optic nerves and the retinas, and cataracts had formed, too. It seemed to me that sorting all that out was going to be a daunting task. Also, somewhere deep down, I was beginning to feel that to seek healing for my blindness was to admit that, as a blind person, I had failed. I was embarrassed, too, that my friends were devoting so much time to me.

Nothing, however, would put them off. They were convinced that this was what they had to do, and they were determined to go through with it. Members of a church in Derby became involved, although they did not meet with us. I felt strongly that I had done nothing to deserve all this love and concern, and really wished it had happened to someone else. My friends had nothing to gain from this, and most of them would not thank me for mentioning their names. I suppose another reason for my discomfiture was that I was afraid that I might be thought of as a religious crank. I do not consider myself to be 'religious' in the way that word is so often used. I have a deep faith, but it has always been a private matter, and my feet, I like to think, have always been firmly planted on the ground.

The celebration dinner on my birthday, in February, was to have more far-reaching effects than any of us could then have imagined. The drama of the occasion itself was shattering enough – the episode needed no epilogue, one might have thought.

Ian and I chose a friendly restaurant where we had

eaten several times. I had a new dress, a new hairstyle, and had gone to town with the make-up. Whether I looked it or not, I felt a million dollars. The meal was good, and so was the wine. The soft music enhanced the general atmosphere of cosiness. The world felt like a good place to be in, and I was enjoying pretending to myself that this was the way we ate and lived every day of the week.

During the first course I began to feel quite strange. Everything was floating away. I was only about half-way down the first glass of wine, but slowed up, just in case. Two mouthfuls into the delicious sweet, and the swimming sensation became so bad that I couldn't keep quiet about it any longer. The conversation was just not reaching my brain. As I leaned my head against the wall beside me, it became obvious to the others that I felt ill.

At first they teased, telling me I'd had too much to drink and would have to learn to take it. When Ian managed to lift his eyes from his sweet – always the favourite course for him – he was shocked into instant action. Apparently, I had gone a horrid shade of grey, and my face was strangely twisted.

I don't remember much more about it. Rain on my face told me that I was still alive, for I do remember, at one stage, quite calmly accepting the fact that I was making a sudden and untimely departure from this world. The ambulance men were kind and reassuring, and so were the night staff in the casualty department of the Infirmary to which I was taken.

I spent a couple of hours there, wired up to a gadget that bleeped out information about the condition of my heart to all those who wished to know and were able to interpret its findings. I was attacked, in a very gentle and civilized manner, with hammers. The doctor seemed enormously gratified when my left foot shot into the air, nearly knocking her off her own feet, after the first of these attacks. There were blood tests and innumerable questions. No stone was left unturned. By this time, I felt almost completely well again, and told them so, thinking longingly of the uneaten sweet and the coffee which hadn't even materialized, owing to my hasty departure. Goodness, I'd have given them a hefty donation towards the upkeep of their bleeping heart monitor in exchange for a cup of something hot.

After what seemed an eternity, Ian was allowed back in. The doctor explained that I had suffered neither a heart attack nor a stroke. Well, that was reassuring news. Apparently, some people have a tendency, if they eat a large meal after more or less fasting all day, to have the sort of attack I had suffered.

By this time, I could think only of the boys at home. The lady who had sat with them would have gone home by now, and if one of them woke up and looked at his watch, he'd be worried to find us not there. I was told that I had to wait until the duty doctor discharged me, and he was busy, just then, on one of the wards, but wouldn't be too long.

'Come on, let's go,' I urged, sitting up, and putting my feet over the trolley's side. I am surprised that I didn't immediately suffer a genuine heart attack. I had not realized that I was still wired up to the garrulous machine, and it began to shout all sorts of bits of information to the whole casualty department, at the top of its voice and at such speed that I thought it might need to avail itself of its own services if it didn't soon calm down.

I lay down quickly, and tried to pretend that the short disturbance had had nothing to do with me. Eventually the doctor arrived. He studied the notes on my case, and then stunned me by asking: 'How long have you had that squint?' The hair-do, the evening-style make-up, the new red dress, were all perhaps a little dishevelled by now, but surely he should have noticed them first. I had always known that my right eye had a tendency to wander out into the corner, but I think this was the first time it had actually been referred to as 'a squint', which, indeed, is exactly what it was. I felt mortified, although I bear him no grudge, for he did me an enormous favour that night.

'Well,' I told Ian on the way home, 'there's one thing that's certain – I'm going to have that eye sorted out as soon as possible. An eye specialist I saw some years ago suggested that I should have it done for cosmetic reasons, but I didn't take him up on it. I can't think why on earth I didn't, but I shan't mess about any longer.' As it happened, the specialist concerned had moved away and as the days went by the incident went temporarily out of my mind.

CHAPTER 15

'I Can See'

The air outside our back door was heavy with the scent of broom, and the boys remarked that the bluetits were flitting in and out of a little hole in the stone wall that divides two levels of the garden. They had built there the previous year, too. I love to think that they are able to make a safe home in our garden. The pungent smell of broom and the joyous hymn of praise with which the blackbird outside our bedroom window was beginning to fill the dawn air told me that spring had jumped out of bed, and had danced light-footed into our garden and across the fields.

Week by week, my friends in the healing group continued to meet. Some of them had hoped and prayed for more years than I had known. To my shame I had to admit, if only to myself, that most of the time I was certain my faith did not match theirs. Oh, yes, I certainly believed that God could do anything – *everything*! But I really could not imagine myself ever being able to see. One night, I said in my prayers, 'O God, if you don't make me see soon, I'm going to have to pretend. They're all going to be so disappointed, and I shall feel that I've let them down.' In spite of me, they carried on.

One lunchtime Wendy, my social worker, and I were having a cup of coffee during one of her routine visits. Something had brought the subject of the squint into my mind. In the course of the conversation, the name of a Jordanian eye specialist was mentioned, but only more or less in passing. That night I mentioned him to Ian, but again only casually, just to make conversation, really. He surprised me by immediately saying that he felt I should make an appointment to see him as soon as possible. There was such a note of urgency in his voice that I rang Wendy next day, and she promised to contact the specialist as soon as he returned to England. Apparently he spends several months of each year abroad.

An appointment was made for me to see the specialist on a Friday afternoon in the middle of July. At the time, and looking back now, it was one of the strangest days I can remember, but I cannot explain why there was such an unnatural, dream-like quality about everything that happened.

It was one of the few really hot days of the summer. Victor and I travelled into Derby on the bus. I was so proud of him that day. I don't think we had been to Derby together for at least a year, but he wove our way, in and out, between the considerable crowds and had remembered all the road crossings. He took the fairly complicated shopping precinct in his stride, and he had remembered the shop where a year earlier I had bought duvet covers and curtains. We paid it another visit and bought new curtains for Ben's room.

The air was oppressive. I felt stifled in the crowded shopping precinct, and dreadfully churned up inside. I went into Woolworth's for a cup of coffee, as I had about twenty minutes to fill before meeting Ian at two o'clock. In the bustling self-service cafeteria I told Victor 'Find the counter'. He did so and an assistant carried my coffee and showed me to a table. After fiddling with the sealed foil top of the tiny container of cream, my fingers were sticky, so I put out my hand to try to locate a serviette. To my horror and disgust, I put my fingers into an un-emptied ashtray. I felt angry. It is those little things, to which people would normally hardly give a thought, that can be so frustrating to disabled people. You learn to cope with the big things in life – they are a part of daily living, so you get on and tackle them – but to stick your fingers into a dirty ashtray, particularly when you are going somewhere special and want to arrive looking and feeling your best, seems so unnecessary and stupid.

I asked a lady on the next table where the serviettes were. Bless her, she handed me instead a little sachet with a fresh-smelling damp tissue. In spite of having enough to do, I would have thought, shopping with a baby and a toddler, she said she would go with me to the door, as the place was crowded and people were walking about with trays of hot food. My temporary anger melted as Victor and I followed her to the door. I thanked her, and told her that if she had given me a hundred pounds I would not have been as grateful as I had been for that little wet tissue.

When Ian and I arrived at the consultant's house, his gentle wife took us upstairs. There was such a calm, cool atmosphere there that I relaxed, and began to feel more at peace inside. The air was sweet with the scent of roses, and the busy world outside seemed to have melted away. As soon as I met Mr Salem, I knew that I was going to hear something special that day.

Without hesitation, he told me that a simple operation could straighten the squint. I then broached the subject of the cataracts. There followed a very thorough examination. I felt tense again. After what seemed to me an interminable length of time, I heard him saying, 'Part of your optic nerve is healthy. I am willing to remove the cataracts. You have nothing to lose.'

The whole world seemed to whizz round and round me at top speed. I felt like a tiny pin-point in the centre of a huge, spinning wheel. I asked him to say it again. The words, 'You have nothing to lose', suddenly assumed fantastic proportions, zooming towards me, and then

receding into the distance so that they almost faded
away.

Now Mr Salem was speaking again. He told me that the
simple operation would last for forty-five minutes, that I
would be in hospital for a week, and that I would have to
convalesce for six weeks. He went on to say that it could be
done at the end of July or the end of October, as during
August and September he would again be out of the
country. In a state of utter confusion, I asked if I might
phone him within the next day or two, when I had had time
to sort out domestic arrangements. He agreed, and we left.

Cataract surgery is a completely routine operation
these days. The lens of the eye, which has become
opaque, is removed and a plastic lens implanted – a great
improvement on the earlier method, which necessitated
a substitute lens being built into the patient's spectacles.
In my case, the unknown quantity was how much vision
might be restored by this technique. Surgery cannot, of
course, replace a partially atrophied retina or optic nerve
and there was no doubt that mine were affected: no one
could tell how seriously until after the operation.

My mind was in complete and utter confusion. My
brain felt as though it were attached to no other part of
me, and I had an overwhelming desire to cry. It sounds
ridiculous. I had been offered a tiny glimmer of hope –
just the tiniest chance of regaining some sight. I should
have been walking on air, and instead I was sitting head
down, a huge wave of depression curling itself round
and round me like some venomous snake.

Ian told me straightaway that he thought I should
settle for the end of July, although I argued that that
would interfere with our holiday in Wales. He told me
some time later that he had been certain that if I had
decided on October I would not have gone through with
it. I'm sure he was right.

Why did I react in such a strange way? Although I had not expected to be offered any hope at all of regaining any sight, I was suddenly afraid that if I had an operation, and it was unsuccessful, I would not be able to face the cruel disappointment.

On the following Monday I thanked my friends for the encouragement of their faith; and the week after that, I was able to tell them, with complete honesty, that at last my faith matched theirs. It seemed significant, too, that my children never once said 'If Mum can see', but always 'When Mum can see'. Never, once, from then on did I doubt the outcome of the operation.

Nevertheless, I felt bleak as, sitting alone by the bed in the large ophthalmic ward, I heard Ian's footsteps receding further and further from me. When the other patients came back from lunch in the dayroom, they were obviously a lively group, but it was hours before anyone spoke to me. Later that evening they told me laughingly that they had all made overtures to me, in the form of waves, smiles, and nods, but when I failed to respond, they had come to the conclusion that I was 'stuck up' and wanted to be left alone. It wasn't until later that afternoon, when they had seen a nurse leading me by the arm as I went upstairs for routine tests, that they had realized I could not see at all. After that, I became one of them, and everyone was friendly and kind.

There was no need to have worried about Monday, the day on which the operation was performed. The hospital staff were so sensitive, and laughed at us so much in our unflattering gowns and funny paper hats that, joining in the fun, I hardly had time to think about my fears.

Just before two o'clock, I was wheeled off to the operating theatre, and there were the anaesthetist and his staff, who had introduced themselves on the ward that morning. It was comforting to know who they were, to have had time to chat briefly with them. Someone, I think it was the anaesthetist, having explained about the injection I would receive, then said, 'Think of something pleasant, and you'll dream about it during your operation.' I remembered a big, old-fashioned picture that had hung in our living-room when I was a small child. It was a picture of a child in bed, with a very white, conventional-looking angel standing with its wings spread over the cot. As a small child I had hated the dark, and often before I went to sleep, when 'downstairs' seemed almost as though it didn't exist, I would think of that angel in the picture and feel safe. So I decided then, just as the needle went into my hand, that I would think of angels. I don't remember dreaming of anything, but I was certainly not at all afraid.

When I woke up, the nursing staff were so kind – nothing seemed to be too much trouble for them – but, oh, how I wished Ian could be there. I didn't want him to talk to me or do anything for me, just to hold my hand so that I would know he was there, just as he had been through the long hours when the babies were being born, and the day when I had been told that Neana was not going to be able to work any longer, and the day when I had held Dana in my arms for the last time.

All at once it was Tuesday morning. The familiar voices of nurses I had now known for three days told me that they were going to get me out of bed and take me to the dayroom for breakfast. For me, of course, it was no hardship eating my breakfast with the large dressing covering my eye. I had eaten my food for years without seeing it.

And then, the half-dreaded, half-longed-for moment had arrived. As I walked, with the same two nurses who had got me out of bed, into the treatment room to have the dressing removed, it was just as though an automatic

switch in my brain had flipped and not a single thought
seemed to be capable of birth, let alone growth. As I
waited for the truth to be uncovered, my mind was
completely numb. The atmosphere in that small room
was charged with electricity – much like those moments
just before a thunderstorm, when you wonder why the
silence is so loud and realize that all the birds have
stopped singing. No one was singing just then.

Slowly, I lifted my head. I do not know what I had
expected. I think, perhaps, I had not dared to expect
anything – just hoped, perhaps, for something. I saw a
bright, horizontal light, and then, turning my head to the
right, three more bright lights, but these were vertical.

'What can you see?' one of the nurses asked, tenta-
tively. I told her about the lights. I could tell she was
puzzled, and my heart began to thud.

Turning my head again, to the left this time, something
really bright glinted there. I pointed to it, and the feeling
of relief in the room was tangible. I had pointed to the
silver buckle on the other nurse's uniform belt. But what
of those mysterious horizontal and vertical lights? Then,
suddenly, the truth dawned. The former was the white
frame across the top of the door, and the latter three
white bottles standing on the brown shelf of a cupboard.
To me, anything light took on an overwhelming
brightness.

Looking down, I saw several bright shafts of light, all
pointing the same way, with deep, deep shadows
between them. I was puzzled: what could this be, so near
to me, yet looking quite unlike anything to which I could
put a name? I moved my hand, involuntarily, and several
of the bright shafts disappeared – I had been looking at
my fingers.

Our hearts settled to their normal rate, except for, in
mine, a strange fluttering. We walked back into the

dayroom. I told them all, 'I can see.' We wept silent, grateful tears.

For a while, nothing looked like anything that I could interpret. A nurse and I walked up the ward. I could see that the floor was light, but every now and again my eye was aware of something completely dark there. In answer to my question, I was told that these were black tiles, set at random among the light ones. With squeals of joy, I went round my part of the ward 'spotting the black tile'. It seems crazy that such a simple thing could give so much pleasure. The nurse who was with me at the time said that she had never realized there could be so much poetry in a black tile – nor had I!

At first, as I dared to look at the people around me, I felt mixed up and almost afraid. None of their features seemed to be in the right places. All the eyes looked as though they were very near the tops of the heads, and it was some time before I could locate the noses. I didn't like it at all when people smiled, or opened their mouths wide. Faces seemed, at first, to have a menacing look about them. Their mouths looked so dark, and pulled themselves into grotesque shapes. Bit by bit, though, it all began to fall into place. The faces of some of the nurses took much longer to make out than others, and then we realized that these were the ones with blond hair. Dark hair gave definite frame to the face, making it possible for me to focus upon it more easily.

Then one of the nurses walked up the middle of the ward. I listened to her footsteps, and watched her. I began to laugh and laugh. Her legs didn't seem to belong to her body at all. They looked like something that hung from beneath her skirt, and made strange scissor-like movements as they dangled there. I am still amazed by people's legs as I watch them walking along the pavement in front of me. I can't really explain why. I am just fascinated by the way in which they move, and the feet at the bottom still make me laugh.

As the day went on, facial features began to form some sort of ordered pattern, and then the edge of a window-sill near my bed and the rails of the curtains around my bed came more sharply into view. All the time I kept seeing more and more things that had to be identified for me. I had forgotten all about drain-pipes on the outside walls of buildings. I had no idea that those long, sleek metallic shapes outside the window were cars. How on earth was one to sort out the front from the back? At first I imagined that they were aeroplanes, except that I knew they couldn't be. Goodness, what would the world be throwing at my brain next?

In fact the world, determined to join in with the fun, began laughingly to throw handfuls and handfuls of objects my way. What on earth was that straight line that kept landing right across my dinner when I was trying to eat it? 'That's your knife,' a nurse explained. Heavens, I reminded myself of the children when they were tiny – 'What's that? What's that?' at almost every move we made.

That afternoon I heard Ian's footsteps coming up the ward. So many times I had listened for those footsteps, and here they were, coming closer, and then his hand took hold of mine. And there he was, and I was looking at him – looking at my own husband, for the very first time. I had always thought about him, with his dark hair and dark eyes, and somehow knew what he would look like: I wasn't really surprised. I was surprised, though, when suddenly I became aware that I was looking straight into his eyes, straight at him. My eye, with new sight, had caught his eyes, and he couldn't get away. I held him, almost like a captive there, and he couldn't get away. I have never had that feeling since, but I shall never, never forget it – the first time I caught someone's eye. I am glad it was someone I loved. I think Ian was embarrassed too, by this new experience, for after a few moments he looked away, with a little smile.

It took him a long time to get used to me watching him. Sometimes, in the car, I would watch his hands on the steering wheel, and for months I could sense his discomfiture.

Several dear, close friends came that day to visit me. It was wonderful to see them. They all looked lovely to me. They were all smiling, and their faces looked as though they were filled with light. Smiles, I now realized, do wonderful things to the plainest face. I stared, and stared. I focused so slowly, that I had to stare, and I still do. Probably people who don't understand think me very rude, but I love looking at faces, and so I tend to stare at them still. That day, the first day of my new sight, nobody seemed to care how much I stared at them.

In the evening, Ian brought Adam and Ben to see me. For all these years, I had known them as only a mother can know, sensing every mood, anticipating every reaction. That first sight of them was breathtaking – my breath caught in my chest and couldn't get free for a moment or two. I don't think I shall ever tire of looking at their faces. I love to look at them, watch them. When I go in, now, to waken Ben in the mornings, I stand at the door and look at his dark head on the pillow, and something indescribably, sweetly painful swells up inside me. Adam was fifteen, and Ben was ten, and I had to gather up all those years in my arms, and spin round and round with them all in my arms, spinning through those unseeing years, until we arrived at 'now' and the first ever sight of my two boys.

They were almost unmoved by the situation and hardly questioned me at all. I think perhaps it threatened their security, although I am sure they couldn't have put that into words. Their Mum had never been able to see, and they understood that. For them that was normal, and this situation, a Mum with a completely new dimension, must have been a little alarming.

When it was time for them to go, they all three stood at the end of my bed, the three pairs of dark eyes, all so similar, looking back at me. I shall always carry, in my little box of treasures, the memory of those three lovely pairs of eyes looking, perhaps almost wistfully, at me. And then they were gone. They disappeared and became a blur among all the other things, reverting to the more familiar three pairs of footsteps receding into the distance.

And all the time the laughing old world continued to throw, like handfuls of confetti, one new experience after another. There were more visits, from friends long loved but never seen, and the thrill of witnessing my parents' joy. One thing after another the dear world threw, and they landed beside my bed to be picked up and gazed upon, or wondered at. That was a week full of laughter, and the staff, no matter how busy they were, seemed somehow to manage to stop in their tracks just long enough to answer my newest 'What's that?'

When Mr Salem came on his routine visit, I sensed that even he was startled. 'I prayed to God,' he told me, 'before I started, while I operated, and after the operation I thanked him – I always do.'

CHAPTER 16

Homecoming

On the following Saturday, just four days after the dressings had been removed from my eyes, I went home. No words of thanks were adequate to express my gratitude to every one of the staff and patients in the ophthalmic ward of the Infirmary for their skill, patience and encouragement. I think they understood that I felt more than I could say.

As we covered the nine miles or so between the hospital and home, I could see all kinds of things to which, like the drainpipes on the hospital walls, I had given no thought for years. I was amazed to see tall vertical lines flashing by, and to learn that these were lamp-posts and telegraph poles. For years I had per-ceived these as a temporary blocking out of the sound of clear space. I certainly had given no thought to the part which went on up, above my head, into the air. If I had been aware of street lamps at all, it would have been merely as something to be avoided, but since the dogs had taken care of that for so many years, I suppose I had more or less forgotten about them.

The white line in the middle of the road fascinated me: I loved watching the way it seemed to run on ahead, as though it was showing us the way, going round the bends in the road just seconds before we got there. Sometimes it was joined by another line, running along close beside it, and then the two would merge into one again.

For years I hated car journeys. I was a slightly nervous passenger and was impatient, sitting there with the engine droning on, sometimes for hours, aware of how much time I was wasting. Suddenly I realized that this nine-mile stretch of road, along which I had been driven hundreds of times, was like a voyage into an unknown land. Never again, I thought, as we passed one thing after another, never again shall I be glad when a journey is over.

We arrived at the house. I had not expected the sudden turn in the path, the unexpected corner around which I could not see, for the tall, thickly-leafed trees hid what was ahead. But I could see the dark and pale tones of leaves alongside each other on the same branch. And I was filled with wonder at the beauty of the bark on the thick trunks as the low sunlight glanced across them, creating exquisite contrasts of light and deep shadow.

As we went indoors I didn't think about looking, for the familiar sounds and smells took over. This was my home, with the rubber mat at the front door which grabs your foot if you're wearing high heels. Then across the ridge at the door, and you step on to the soft carpet. Just after you've closed the front door, there's a narrow bit between the stairs and a chest of drawers where you have to concentrate so that you don't catch yourself on the corner of the piece of furniture.

I heard the familiar click of the living-room door opening, and they were there, Martin and Victor, all legs and mouths; Victor squeaking with pleasure, tumbling over himself with excitement, Martin standing gently by, waiting for the moment when I would find him and stroke his domed old head. Then I saw them. I saw, for the very first time, the two pairs of gentle dark eyes that for so many years had taken the place of my eyes whenever I went out alone – but never alone; and not for the first time tears filled my eyes. I had had no idea that those two gentle, trusting faces looking up at me would tug with such strength at my heart-strings. I had always known that my dogs were beautiful. Everyone had told them, and me, how handsome they were, but the magnetic effect their gentle eyes had upon me was astounding.

My home, too, every inch of which I knew by heart, took on a new dimension. I had always thought of the furnishings in our living-room as having quiet, gentle colours and patterns but, as I looked during those first few minutes, the pattern on the carpet and cushions seemed to zoom towards me shouting, 'We're here! You didn't know we were big and noisy like this, did you?' The buttons on the back of the settee looked as though they had been dropped to the bottom of deep, deep wells. I had to touch them with my fingers, to convince myself that it was the same piece of furniture that had been there when I had left, just a week ago. I was puzzled when I looked towards the fireplace by the deep, dark shadows that criss-crossed irregularly all over it – my fingers told me that the dark lines were the crevices between the stones.

The house was full of beautiful flowers, bouquets and basketfuls in every room. They were so lovely, so fragile, quietly welcoming me to this old-new home I thought I had known so well. I couldn't believe that all those flowers had been sent for me, by family and friends who wanted to tell me how glad they were for me. I was deeply moved by their love and kindness.

One thing that still bothered me was the monochrome world I was living in. Everything was in shades of black, white and grey. Where had the colours gone? For years, whenever colours had been mentioned, I had been able to see them clearly in my mind's eye, but whatever I looked at with my real eyes had no colour at all. The other strange thing was that even though I could see things fairly clearly, I could not identify them until I touched them. Even a knife, the sort we had been using at every meal for years, lying on the kitchen table, mystified me until touching it solved the puzzle.

In the euphoria of those first heady days in hospital, I had told one of the nurses that I wanted to stand on a mountain-top and tell the whole world I could see. Not that I wanted the world to know about me – I simply wanted to share this wonderful thing with everybody: sight was such a miracle that everyone should be given an opportunity to share the glory of it. It wasn't *my* sight, just the concept of seeing that was so marvellous: I thought I would never want to think or talk about anything else again.

On the evening after my dressings had been removed, the headline of one of our local newspapers read, in enormous letters, 'I CAN SEE'. Slowly I spelled them out. (I had never forgotten the shapes of capital letters, although I was soon to discover that I was quite incapable of reading what I call 'curly writing'.) 'I CAN SEE', and I read it, and it was about me. But it didn't seem to be about me as a person, but about this unique sense, which has nothing to do with touching, and hearing, and smelling.

By the next day the media had got hold of the story, and I agreed to be interviewed by reporters and a local TV station. In retrospect I wonder whether it would have been better if everything had been kept quiet, for life would have been quieter and there would have been more opportunity to learn to use this new sight. At the time it seemed that this was the mountain-top I had wished for and, it having been put there, the most logical thing to do was to get up on it and let whoever was listening hear the good news.

About half an hour after I got home from the hospital, a reporter from one of the daily newspapers arrived wanting to do an article about my homecoming. He stood at the window and commented on the magnificent view. Almost everyone coming into that room for the first time remarks on the view. I have heard it described time and time again – the whole panorama of Belper, with its houses sprawling up the hillside, the tower and the spire of the two churches on the other side of the valley, factories, schools, and beautiful open countryside. People have stood there at the window, picking out the houses of people they know, a mile or more away from us. I never really understood it, but I knew it all by heart. I knew, too, about the nearer things, down in the valley – the cotton mill with its chimney pointing heavenward like some great work-blackened finger, the lights in its many windows telling us how many people were working there at night. Just beside it the river flows, picking up the reflection of the main road's lights at night. There is a splendid view of the river gardens beside the mill, with the lovely old bandstand where a band plays every Sunday evening through the summer months, and families stroll beside the river or sit on the seats and listen to the music unaware, probably, that they are observed by us, up on the hill.

I hadn't realized that through the years I had built up my own semi-visual picture of all this. And I was not prepared for the shock when the reporter asked, 'What do you think of this wonderful view?'

I looked and was silent.

'Can you see the fire station's red doors?' he went on, 'and the churches over there?'

All so immediately obvious to him, with his perfect vision which, after years of daily use, can take in everything, however unfamiliar, at a glance. I couldn't explain to him that the higgledy-piggledy lumps and bumps in various shades of black, white and grey meant nothing to me and bore no relation to the beautiful picture in my mind's eye. I think it was probably then that I realized that this wonderful new sight, which had intoxicated me from the moment the dressings had been removed, was not like other people's. That did not make it any less wonderful to me, but I think I realized then that it was going to present its own particular problems for other people as well as for me.

At night, when the street lamps came on, I forgot all about not being able to interpret the lumps and bumps. There, scattered all over the darkness, were dozens and dozens of lights, starting way below the level of our window, and rising in a great formless scatter, higher and higher into the sky. What a stunning sight! No common street lamps these. They assumed the dimensions of mystic sentinels, valiant, upright and brave, guarding the dark hillside with flaming swords held aloft. Or was it perhaps an aged and wise monarch, bent and bowed with antiquity, whose splendour lived on in his flashing eyes and the great dark cloak, thrown over his time-hunched shoulders, his one-time splendour preserved in the sparkling, twinkling, flaming of that jewel-bespangled cloak?

Even without these fanciful thoughts, what I saw that first night at home could not have failed to astound me. Never had I imagined the valley so deep and the hills so high. I stood and gazed, almost hypnotized by this awesome sight. I know that I shall never tire of it. I must have spent hours since then, just gazing into the night, enchanted by those lights that have shone there all these years without my knowing it. When I wake up in the night, I almost always sit up, just to snatch another look at those ever-watchful sentinels of the night.

In those early days I would sit for hours on the edge of my bed looking out of the front window at the houses across the road. It was easy to make out the line of the house-tops and, after a while, the shape of the chimneys standing up. One day I called Ian to show him some large black and white strips on the sides of some of the houses. He could make no sense at all of what I had described, and it was not very helpful that, at that time, I seemed to be incapable of pointing in the direction that I was looking: there seemed to be no co-ordination between eye and hand. It suddenly dawned upon him that I was looking at the windows of the house – the white stripes were their frames and the black stripes the glass. Sometimes, I learnt, the people who live across the road would wave to me, but I wasn't able to see them. It must have been disconcerting for them, seeing me sitting there hour after hour, looking and looking, but not knowing how much I could see, or what I was looking at.

Another day, becoming aware of something white, sticking straight up in the air just beside the house across the road, I set poor Ian another brain-teaser. This one took even longer to sort out, and I became thoroughly frustrated – it looked so clear and obvious to me. By this time Ian had become quite expert at interpreting my descriptions, but there was nothing white that stuck up in the air beside the house across the road. It wasn't until the next day, when I identified a shape like a car on it, that we realized it was the drive. It still didn't look flat to me, even after I knew what it was. In those early days I appeared to have no sense whatsoever of perspective.

Once I had located the mill chimney, about a week after arriving home, that became a special landmark, by which I judged and measured everything. It can be seen from so many parts of the town and surrounding countryside that, for me at any rate, it has something of the quality and value of a compass or a lighthouse to a sailor.

I became used to the fact that I could see much better on some days than on others, depending on the quality of the light or even on my own state of physical or mental well-being. One morning, however, Ian brought me a cup of tea and knew immediately that something was wrong. He said my face looked bleak and frightened. I could hardly form the words to tell him that I couldn't see the houses across the road. He chuckled and went quickly to the other side of the bed to pull back the curtains, and there they were: roofs, chimneys, stripey windows – and the drive, which by now had taken up its rightful position on the ground. I hadn't realized until that moment how much this imperfect, crazy sort of sight meant to me, and how fearful I was that something might go wrong. Always, since that day, Ian warns me if it is misty and even he can't see the mill chimney or the horizon.

During the next days and weeks the letters and flowers continued to arrive. The simple message of each card and letter moved me deeply. I was always astonished that people had bothered to write to me, many of whom did not know me at all. There were dozens of letters from past pupils and colleagues, each with some precious memory of days gone by. They will never know what their letters meant to me.

A letter came from a Mr Arthur Jones, who had been the chaplain at St Gabriel's, my teacher training college. Suddenly, although he had not mentioned it, a memory was awakened in my mind. All those years ago, before I knew anything about the Church's ministry of healing, and when I would not even have admitted to myself that I really believed in such things or had any need of them, he asked if I would agree to a short service in which I would be anointed with oil. Not wishing to cause offence, I had agreed. At the time I remember being just a little disappointed because, after the ceremony, I felt no different. However, recalling it all, I knew that in spite of my lack of understanding at the time it had been important, because someone had been courageous enough to show, in public, that he believed in the power of prayer.

CHAPTER 17

Learning to See

Two weeks after coming home, I saw for the first time the church where, more than sixteen years before, Ian and I had been married, and which I had attended regularly for the past eleven years and where I had sung in the choir for five or six of those years. My feet were familiar with every inch of St Peter's. The doormat inside the porch always seemed a little bit thicker than I remembered it. There were two metal carpet strips – one at the sliding glass doors between the west end and the nave and another one a step or two further on. I never quite understood about that, and never failed to be surprised when my foot touched the hard surface of the second.

At one point, half-way down the aisle, if I was wearing high-heeled shoes the carpet seemed to grab at one of them. Sometimes, particularly if there had been a wedding the day before, I would feel something brushing gently against my arm: I discovered there were small arrangements of flowers in holders at the end of each pew. Then the person I was walking with would press my arm slightly, and I knew I was at the chancel steps; the carpet surface changed and became softer and deeper. Another nudge, and it was time to bow my head at the step to the sanctuary and turn off to the left, off the carpet, and hear my heels clicking on the marble slabs. One small step up and the sound changed, became softer and very hollow-sounding, as we slid into our places in the choir-stalls. I loved the rough-smooth feel of the wood of the choir-stalls, with its rather open-grained texture. It had a warm, friendly feel to it, almost like something that was not inanimate at all. The smell, too, has a sort of timelessness about it, as though you had been born with it in your nostrils: a mish-mash of old books, damp, and wax polish, it belongs exclusively to Sunday.

What the church looks like, inside and out, had been described to me many times, but as I stood there that first Sunday, actually seeing it for myself, I realized, not for the first time, that there are some things no words can adequately describe. I knew that the roof, inside, was red, and that embroidered and appliquéd banners made by members of the congregation hung from the balcony which ran round three sides of the church, and I knew there were stained-glass windows. What I had not known until that first moment was how gentle fingers of light slant through those windows and seem to caress the old wood of the pews, leaving here and there, along the length of each, small pools of light, which glowed with a soft, lustrous glow, rather like a moonstone I have. I didn't know what to look at first – there was so much to see. Yes, up there, those must be the banners, and that very light expanse, on which they hung, that must be the front of the balcony. I couldn't really make much of the banners. Each looked like a jumble of shapes in different shades of grey and white and black.

Looking up, I saw that the ceiling was dark, and assumed that this must be the red part. I was surprised, though, that the whole lot was criss-crossed with white strips – probably wood – which divided it into squares. To the left, near the front, something stuck up into the air. It looked pointed at the top. I presumed that this was some sort of musical instrument which had been propped up against something, and, noticing it still there on several subsequent Sundays, just had to go at last and investigate. My tethered instrument turned out to be the wooden top of the font.

It was fascinating to watch the members of the congregation, as they stood there in their rows, slanting away from me. Every head was bowed at a similar angle as they sang the hymns and songs, bending over the words in the books. I don't know why that fascinated me so. Looking towards the front, there was the altar, before which Ian and I had knelt on our wedding day, all those years before, and where, countless times, I had knelt to receive communion; now it had some sort of substance, if perhaps a little dreamlike. The gentle light gleamed quietly on the metal of the cross, and I could see the straight, vertical lines which must be candlesticks and candles. The jumbled-looking shapes which I could not then interpret on either side of the cross were flowers, I found out later.

At that time I still had to move my head quite a lot to look at things. What an odd figure I must have been, that first Sunday, sitting there turning my head this way and that, looking up at the ceiling, trying to count the squares made by the criss-crosses of wood. It hadn't really registered in my mind, either, that other people could see me – far more clearly, in fact, than I could see them – and that it is not very usual to sit twisting your head, and sometimes your whole body, this way and that, however much you might want to see something.

I had much to thank God for, that day, and had never sung with more feeling the refrain of each verse of the hymn 'How Great Thou Art'. And yet, even as I sang, dreadful feelings of guilt clutched at me and gnawed away, deep down inside. Why me? I'm not particularly good; I have a dreadful temper at times; I often grumble and I'm not always grateful for life's blessings. Why me? I could only conclude that there are some things to which we shall probably never know the answers on this side of the grave.

* * *

By now it was clear to me that there was no question of Victor becoming redundant. In familiar surroundings my sight was very useful indeed. I can often see obstacles in my way and can quite often make out steps. I can look at a house and distinguish the door from the window. I can see where the doors into shops are, and where road crossings are. I can even see the little button you have to press to stop the traffic at pelican crossings. All of these things are tremendously useful, and I sometimes find myself wondering, even after this short time, how on earth I managed some things when I couldn't see at all. But, like most blind people, I didn't stop to wonder how I was managing but just got on and managed.

I had always noticed a few places where Victor habitually slowed down and sometimes even stopped. Finding no reason why he did this, and being unable to get a satisfactory answer from people who could see, I could only assume that he had some private reason of his own. The answer to my questions, however, soon became quite apparent. At two of the points where he appears to hesitate, and at which his hesitation had often given rise to a feeling of irritation in me, the pavements have a very uneven, broken surface. In two more places where my conscientious guide slows down, after it has rained there are enormous puddles, which take a long time to dry up. I had never known about these problem areas simply because Victor had coped with them so efficiently. I can only assume that sighted people had not been able to answer my questions because they tend not to notice the things that they see regularly. To me, seeing them for the first time, the pot-holes seemed menacing, and the drains that I noticed as I stepped up kerbs made me think of mouths with bared teeth, which might open and gobble me up as I passed them.

I had, of course, always been aware of the traffic

roaring by on the main road along which we walk into town. I hadn't realized, though, the terrific height of the lorries that passed us. Sometimes cars would look as though they were driving straight towards me, because at first I didn't understand about bends in the road, and how they alter the appearance of things. It is great fun watching other pedestrians walking along in front of me. When they are at a distance I see them quite plainly. If a person is wearing trousers I try to work out by the walk whether it is a man or a woman, and whether the thing alongside is a bag or a dog. Doorways on the other side of the road are often more visible to me than those on the side on which I am walking, and so are the displays in shop windows.

I felt something of a fraud walking up the main shopping street with a guide dog, and yet being able to look across the road and read the names above shops. It was a relief when a trainer came from Leamington Spa and explained that many people who appear to have a considerable amount of vision would be unsafe in today's crowd and traffic conditions without a dog or some other aid to mobility. Noticing how I flinched as I saw people coming towards me from all angles, the trainer spent considerable time showing me how to use my new sight to help Victor instead of confusing him. After his visit I felt much more positive.

Our local supermarket was almost as familiar to me as my own home. Each week Victor and I would walk round with one of the assistants. I could recite the contents of each stand as we progressed along the various aisles. The assistant would put the items I named into the trolley and pack them into a box at the check-out when I paid for them, leaving the box of groceries for Ian to pick up on his way home in the car. On the first occasion after my operation, I was looking forward to our trip to the

supermarket. I had been very touched when, after I came
out of hospital, some of the supermarket staff had
brought me the most beautiful bouquet of flowers. They
had requested a record for me on Radio Derby, too. Ever
since, 'The first time ever I saw your face' brings a great
lump into my throat. That is so typical of the warm-
heartedness of our local people.

As Victor and I entered the store, I became immediately aware of what seemed like hundreds of dazzling
lights. They looked enormous and seemed to be so low
that I felt as though I could have reached up and touched
them. As I stood there waiting for Jackie, who used to
help me at that time, I felt as though these lights were
coming closer and closer, bearing down upon me like
fiery monsters that would consume me with their
brilliant, hot breath. I was relieved when Jackie arrived
with the trolley. Through the turnstile, the ceiling was
higher and the bright monsters at a safer distance. 'What
biscuits are you having this week?' was always Jackie's
first question. But I wasn't paying attention. I heard her,
but answered the familiar questions mechanically.

As we walked along the aisles, I saw the shelves
packed with tins, jars, packets, looming up into the air
like great, garish giants, lifting their heads towards the
fiery monsters in the ceiling. The dozens and dozens of
labels on the goods towering above me on the shelves
made weird patterns, that zig-zagged about as though
they were alive. I almost cowered as we moved along the
aisles, half-fearful that the boxes of washing-powder and
cereals and other normally innocuous articles would
sprout arms, with little clutching hands and fingers that
would dart out suddenly and grab at me when I wasn't
watching. Never, as I had stood beside a stand deciding
whether to have baked beans or spaghetti, green or pink
soap, had I imagined that they had been scowling back at

me, so hostile and so huge. I was overwhelmed. I hated it. It was like a really dreadful nightmare.

I didn't go to the supermarket again for several weeks. I didn't feel I could face it yet. But, realizing that I couldn't spend the rest of my life hiding from things I couldn't yet completely understand, I went back a few weeks later. This time, I made a conscious effort to look at individual items on the shelves. Suddenly, I could see a ticket, which announced that something was being sold for forty-five pence. So pleased was I with this progress that I looked around, and there, a little way off, was something I couldn't understand at all. On the side of what looked like a large cardboard box, was a longish word, but it ended with a capital M. 'Whatever is that,' I asked, 'that word with a capital M at the end?' Jackie was obviously puzzled, but as the truth dawned she laughed and laughed. What I had seen was one of the cartons in which packets of Weetabix are packed, but as it had been put on a trolley upside-down, the initial capital 'W' had become the 'M' which I was now studying with such bafflement.

Hardly had the mystery of the capital letter at the end of the word been solved when, looking up, I could see, written in large letters above a counter, the word 'Delicatessen'. As I read it aloud, a new confidence flooded through me, as though somebody had injected it straight into one of my veins. I had read a word above the counter, just as all the other shoppers did. That gave me an immense boost. If I could do that, why shouldn't I have a closer look at some of the other labels? I would have to peer at them closely, because that was the way my eyes worked, but I was sure nobody would mind, or think me strange or freakish. Almost drunk with the new delights of supermarket shopping, I took the trolley and steered it along the aisle until, just before the corner,

Jackie grabbed it from me. I had pushed it dangerously near to a pyramid-shaped display of jam and other preserves. She told me she didn't fancy spending the rest of the day sweeping up glass.

I could never have believed that shopping in a supermarket could offer so many thrilling experiences. It may seem rather childish to someone who has always been able to do it, but if you have never walked to the checkout alone before, watching the feet of the people in front and making sure you don't run into them with your laden trolley, it presents an enormous challenge, and you have a remarkable sense of achievement when you've done it. I suppose it was something like being a child all over again. I feel tremendously privileged that, at my age, I have been able to experience such joy in ordinary, simple and mundane things, for the very first time.

As, more and more, I had small tastes of the world of people who have sight, I did begin to think differently about myself. I didn't feel superior, but I gained a new sort of self-respect. I do not mean by this that I feel myself in any way a better person than when I couldn't see anything. It's simply different – a glimpse into a different world, of which I never thought I should be a part.

I had not realized, when I uttered those three words 'I can see', that, in spite of the truth of that statement, I had a great deal to learn on the subject. I was to discover that for me seeing would not be an automatic reflex. For one thing, I had, at most, only twenty-five per cent of normal vision, and only in one eye. Then my eyes had not had to do any work for years and I had no idea how to use them properly. At first I moved my whole head to look at an object which was only inches away from whatever I had previously been looking at. When I walked about, I didn't know where to look – whether just in front of my feet, or at the furthest point away from me. I had no idea about scanning. I didn't realize that I could look up or down without actually moving my head. I found that I focused very slowly, so that I needed to use a mixture of hearing and seeing. For instance, if I go into a room and someone is already there, it is more than likely that I will not see him. However, if he speaks to me, I can locate him, as I have done for years, by the direction from which the voice comes and, having located him, I can then see him very clearly.

Because I have a narrow field of vision, owing to damage at the backs of my eyes, I often get a very clear picture of objects which are some distance from me, while those that are nearer are very blurred and indistinct. Hence, when we go into a pub or café, I find that empty chairs on the other side of the room are easily seen, whereas I fumble to find the one to which I am being shown, and which is right beside me. In public places, I have a very clear view of folk sitting several rows in front of me but because of the tunnel effect of my vision, have been known to carry on an animated, even if one-sided conversation with a space immediately beside me which had been occupied by someone who has just moved away. Ian commented one day that I should have been fitted up with extra long arms when I had my lens implants, as I often grumble that I can see his dinner at the other side of the table more clearly than I can see my own.

Eating presented quite a problem in the early days after the operation. Besides using a knife and fork to cut and stab food and convey it to the mouth, people who cannot see use them to locate food on the plate and to check the size of a piece of food before it is raised to the mouth. It is possible to become very neat and efficient at eating in this way, although there were always certain foods I avoided. Lettuce and cress can present embarrassing problems, because you cannot easily tell if you have cut right through the piece you are about to eat until you feel something flapping around your chin. Poultry on the bone can be very awkward to deal with too. Now there was a new problem. Certainly I could see the food on my plate (and didn't like the look of some of it). The problem was the way the knife and fork kept getting in the way of my seeing the food. It was strange actually to see the fork digging its way into a potato, for instance, and the knife come alongside the fork and cut through the potato, dividing it in two.

I remember, one day during the week after I had come out of hospital, scratching about on my plate with my fork because I could quite clearly see several objects there. Ian smiled as he said, 'I shouldn't bother trying to eat that. It's the pattern on the plate.'

Day after day, new experiences presented themselves, and my uninitiated sight had one surprise after another. I was amazed by the line of dirt on my duster, one day after I had had a blitz on the living-room skirting-boards. Another time I cracked three eggs into a glass basin, and was fascinated by the way they formed a sort of triangle lying there, the yolks still whole, in the bottom of the basin. Only gradually did I realize that I could pour a cup of tea without listening for the note the liquid makes when it has reached the top of the cup, or putting my finger over the rim of the cup and pouring until the liquid just touched my fingertip. Now I was able to see the cup filling, but for months I forgot to look.

I looked at everything, the most ordinary things seeming wonderful and special. I looked at bubbles in the bath, the mortar between bricks, the deep crevices in stone walls, the golden fur in the brushes and combs after I had groomed the dogs. Peeling potatoes became less of a chore as, fascinated, I watched the brown peel fall away to reveal the white flesh beneath. I find it far less tedious, too, to locate the eyes of the potatoes and remove them.

Ironing, for a long time, was a revelation. At first I was surprised by the bold designs of the boys' tee-shirts. I hadn't understood that clothes bore all kinds of inscriptions for the whole world to read in letters so large and bold that even I could decipher them without bending down to the ironing board. I was surprised, too, to be able to see creases in clothes so clearly, and was delighted to watch a wrinkled piece of material smooth out miraculously under the ministrations of my hot iron. Now that I didn't have to search out the creases with my left hand, running it along just in front of the point of the iron, I became very much quicker, and didn't feel so tired after a couple of hours of ironing.

There was always something new and exciting to see and learn about. One night, Ian came rushing in, to tell me that there was a hot-air balloon coming over. I ran out into the garden, and although I could hear the roaring that I recognized immediately, I couldn't locate it with my eyes. I became terribly frustrated, hearing it so clearly, but failing to add sight to sound. Ian called Ben out of the house and, bundling us into the car, set off at some speed, following the balloon along country lanes, losing it now and again and then spotting it in the distance. Ian was determined that I should see it, and I hoped that I wouldn't disappoint him. At last we stopped. Across a field, I could clearly see a line of trees. The balloon, now joined by several more, was just beginning to drop down and, suddenly spotting it, I bounced almost as vigorously as the balloon itself as I squeaked, 'I've got it, I've got it.' I don't know what the group of people standing a short distance away thought of me, but I had just seen my first ever hot-air balloon, and didn't care who knew that I thought it very exciting.

And there was the special, beautiful discovery, one day when we were out walking with the dogs. There lay, on the dark earth, a scattered group of something that looked smooth and faintly iridescent. Their beauty, for me, lay in the stark contrast they made, lying there as though some careless fairy creature had emptied its pockets as it skipped by, leaving a little handful of treasures behind. They were only pebbles, when I bent down and touched them to discover their identity – only ordinary pebbles, but they didn't look ordinary to me. The little brown pony with a white blaze down his face, and the herd of cows making snuffly noises as they crowded to the gate, all looked as though they had come specially to let me see their soft, sweet faces. So often, during those months, as I looked at the faces of small children and gentle beasts, my eyes filled with tears, in response to a new sort of feeling of tenderness these things caused to well up in my heart.

Little by little, as the days went by, I began to understand the things I saw. My brain became more and more efficient at putting together the shapes my eyes could see, and I was able to put names to many of them. Standing at a back window, particularly an upstairs window, I gradually identified one rooftop after another, but was startled when I realized that, even though I was looking right down upon them, they were only in the next road. Only too well did I know about that steep bit of hill between the next road down and ours. How often I had trudged home with a heavy shopping bag, unable to swop hands because the dog must always stay on the left side, where it had been trained to walk. Sometimes I felt that the heavy load would pull me right through the pavement into the earth below, while my heart thudded with the exertion and my feet went mechanically on. No one needed to explain that steep hill to me, but it had never occurred to me that it was almost the height of a house.

The green copper roof of the bandstand never fails to arrest my attention. Of course, at that time it wasn't green to me, but it glows with a lovely iridescent light and looks very round, like the top of an umbrella. On very good days, I can see the point that sticks up in the centre of it. One morning something down near the bandstand came suddenly and unexpectedly alive. It shone and glistened, and appeared to crack up into hundreds of fragments, and then became calm and serene again, but shining as brightly as a mirror. I called one of the boys. 'Oh, it's only the river, Mum,' he said in a matter-of-fact way. Only the river. There can be nothing 'only' about a river that you've looked out upon for ten years, but never seen before. It's a beautiful river.

When a week or two later my brother and his family came to visit us, there was an even more wonderful surprise in store. It was years since I had been out in a rowing boat, and when he suggested it I agreed to go, although, to the horror of my own family, I insisted on wearing a life-jacket. Once we had pulled away from the river gardens, however, it felt as though we were gliding off the edge of the world. The gentle lap-lapping of the oars, the mournful call of water-birds, and the very distant sound of traffic had a soothing effect. And then I saw that trees and bushes were growing upside-down in the dark water. There was a margin of land just beneath its dimpling surface. Far, far down, the sky was bright and dimpling too. The light patches of sky broke up, then re-formed, and the branches of the trees touched the dancing sky, deep down there beneath the water. No wonder musicians have been inspired to weave melody and harmony together in an attempt to recreate the transient beauty of reflections.

I was frustrated by the monochrome world in which I found myself, believing that if I tried a little harder my eyes would break through the veil of dull greys, and the vibrant blues and reds and greens would laugh out at me from their hiding-place. This frustration was intensified by the fact that, upon closing my eyes, and thinking of colours, there they all were, the yellows and pinks and oranges.

My first glimpse of colour occurred after the service one Sunday morning. As I turned my head, there was a sudden bright flash of something – a memory that had no name for a moment. And then I had it. 'Is there something dark blue down there?' I asked my friend Sally, pointing towards a corner of the church. Yes, there is a dark blue curtain. I was delighted, of course, but in spite of this sudden flash of recognition it was several days before I had another similar experience of colour. I was looking for a skirt in my wardrobe, and as I threw an unwanted one on to the bed, the bright cerise colour flashed into my eyes and my brain knew its name. And that's how it was for a long time. There would be a sudden flash of recognition at a time when naming colours was the last thing I was thinking of. Gradually, the dull old blacks and greys were replaced by one tint after another from the great craftsman's palette. Even now, however, if I try too hard, I get colours wrong. If I am not thinking about them, I see them well, but the moment I try to name them I almost invariably get it wrong.

It would be difficult – indeed, well-nigh impossible – to live in a small town like Belper for thirty years and remain anonymous, more especially as I had taught for thirteen years in one of the town's largest schools, thus having been brought into close contact with a large portion of the

community which is now between the ages of twenty-
five and forty. Each of my dogs in turn had won the
admiration and affection of countless townsfolk who,
perhaps, had hardly noticed me. As I have said before,
the people about here are warm, friendly folk who, if
they take to you, really seem to take you to their hearts.
Over the years shopkeepers, bus drivers, traffic wardens
and innumerable others have been wonderfully kind to
me. In the majority of places I am addressed by my
Christian name, and hope it is not too presumptuous of
me to regard these people as friends. I have been told that
when the success of my operation was reported in the
local press there was talk of little else, down in the town. I
am sure that this would have been so whoever I had
been: everybody rejoiced because something good had
happened to someone they knew.

It is difficult for the man in the street to understand that
between perfect sight and total blindness there are many,
many degrees of sight, and that each of these can vary
according to such things as light and a host of other
conditions. A person registered as blind may actually have
a useful degree of residual vision. The subject is complicated, and can give rise to all kinds of misunderstanding.
The first time I went into Belper after my operation, Anne,
who had kindly taken me down in the car, told me that
many of the passers-by were smiling and waving to me.
Although I could easily see the people walking on the other
side of the road, I had no idea who they were and certainly
couldn't see them smiling or waving.

This bothered me. In some strange way I felt that I had
let people down. I felt that I had done something less well
than I might have done, and a sort of grey cloud descended
and began to envelop me. I sat at home for hours after that,
trying to puzzle it all out. To me, it seemed that I could see
so much. I was able to say to the boys, 'Take your feet off

the coffee table', 'Don't read while I'm talking to you', and to friends, 'You've had your hair cut. It suits you.' I had become a part of the world of people who can see, and yet to these very people I appeared to have very little sight indeed. What did it all mean? How did it all work out? Why did I feel such a let-down, sitting there enveloped in the big grey cloud?

I was trying to lose a little weight, but was having difficulty in cutting down on the things I like, all of which, needless to say, are fattening. On the television newsreel a famine, in some faraway country, was being reported. It was dreadful and, as always, moved me deeply. Hearing that these poor people no longer had a clean drinking-water supply, I felt guilty, remembering the countless times I had turned my nose up on being offered a glass of water with a meal. What those dehydrated human beings would have given for just a mouthful or two of water; and to them a slice of bread would have been like a feast. The whole thing, I thought, is relative, and this conclusion slightly eased my feelings of guilt about my comparative affluence.

Then it all fell into place. A person who had always known perfect sight would hardly give a thank-you for what I now have but, for a person who has seen nothing or next to nothing for years, these strange, sometimes even bizarre glimpses into the beauties, and even ordinary things, of the world had become a gluttonous feast of looking.

Pondering further upon the subject, I saw my journey into and out of the world of total blindness as rather like a walk into a long, dark tunnel. As you enter the tunnel, you take a lot of bright daylight in with you. For a long time it is all around you and, even as it gets dimmer and dimmer, your eyes adapt to it, and you can use every last little glimpse of light. Somewhere, deep inside that tunnel, comes the point at which there is no longer any light at all. I think it would be impossible to pin-point that spot with complete accuracy, because by that time you would have learned to interpret the sounds and smells of the tunnel, and started using those to your advantage with such efficiency that your attention would, to some extent, have been diverted from the need for visual images. But you would have taken a host of memories into the tunnel, and they would have a powerful effect upon the way you thought and felt, there in the darkness – the darkness which you didn't actually call by that name and to which, after a while, you probably gave little thought. That is, until you emerged once more into the point where you could see light ahead, and then the thought processes began, and just occasionally, say during a night when you weren't sleeping very well, you would find yourself turning it over and over in your mind, trying to remember exactly what it was like inside the tunnel, but with little success because, when you were in there, you were too preoccupied with moving forward to give it much consideration.

Not long after my operation I attended a conference at a church in Sheffield. I had been there a number of times and, because the floor was carpeted and the chairs of a modern design, I had assumed that the whole interior of the church was modern, too. I could hardly believe my eyes as we went in on this occasion, and I saw pillars and arches, and stained-glass windows. I had to close my eyes and conjure up the picture that had previously been in my mind. Similarly, as the weeks went by, I had all sorts of surprises on meeting people I had known for years. I hadn't realized that I had always constructed a clear visual picture of almost everybody.

One day Sally, whom I had known for a number of years, came to serve me in one of our local shops. I knew her instantly by her voice, but the moment I saw her I blurted out, 'You're not supposed to look like that. You shouldn't have dark hair. You've always been a blonde to me.' She took it in good part, but I had to resist this quick reaction of mine, to comment upon people's looks, as they often assumed I was disappointed, which was rarely the case. Another strange thing was that, if I saw a face before the person spoke to me, I found it difficult to recognize the voice, although it may have been very familiar. That has mostly sorted itself out now, and I am able to identify many people visually. Little wonder, though, that my poor brain didn't know at times how to cope with it all.

The sense of guilt which crept in after I had come down off the high, euphoric cloud took a long time to overcome. I found myself wondering why this had happened to me. I certainly had done nothing to deserve it. There were, I knew, hundreds of people who were far more distressed by their blindness than I had ever been. To lose one's sight in old age, or suddenly as the result of an illness or an accident, must cause terrible pain and grief. This sense of unworthiness plunged me more deeply into a state of depression. My early joy appeared to me then as something rather vulgar and shameful, and I stopped wanting to talk to anyone about the wonderful thing that had happened. I must say here that a number of friends, both blind and partially-sighted, some of whom I'd known for years and others for only a short time, rang or wrote to congratulate me on my good fortune. Two or three even came to see me in hospital. I was very deeply touched by their great-heartedness. One friend, whom I had not seen for years, tried dozens of Taylors on the phone before he tracked me down. He said, 'I'm wildly envious, kid, but if it couldn't happen to me, I'm glad it's happened to you.' Generosity indeed.

CHAPTER 18

Old Places, New Faces

I have always particularly enjoyed teaching first-year children. There is a sort of appealing innocence about them as, smart in their brand-new school uniforms, they try not to betray the fact that they are utterly bewildered by all that there is to learn and remember during those first few days in secondary school. I have often chuckled to myself as, sitting there, hearing my ludicrous threats of the dreadful fates that may befall them if they do not conform to the standards I expect, they are obviously not quite certain how to react. That I am joking is fairly obvious, but that I expect a high standard of good behaviour is obvious too.

First-year pupils, I have found, are keen and enthusiastic, and eager to please. I was delighted, therefore, when I was invited to take the first-year music classes at St Benedict's, at the start of the new term in the September after my operation. I would be filling in once a week for the regular teacher who was on a course throughout that year. At that time the arts subjects were being taught at an annex south of Derby, about sixteen miles from our house. One of the staff kindly offered to pick me up in the morning, and took me back to the main school in the afternoon, where I caught a bus to complete the journey. This felt like real teaching, with plenty of job satisfaction. The frustrating part, often, with supply teaching, is that just as you are building up some sort of relationship with the children, and gaining their confidence, the work comes to an end, and you may never see those children again. I certainly used to feel that I had earned my keep on those Tuesdays, arriving home exhausted, but truly satisfied.

I suppose it was not too odd that, at first, I didn't think of looking across the classroom to see what the children were doing, but continued to rely on the information my other senses gave me. One day, however, I looked across the room and noticed that one boy was still sitting down, after I had asked the class to stand. He was flabbergasted when he realized that I had actually seen him. After that, I found myself using my sight more and more. I think the poor children were utterly confused. Here was a teacher they thought of as being blind, who had a guide dog and needed a bit of help getting around the school, yet had a disconcerting way of suddenly spotting you doing something you might have expected to get away with. I loved the children's frank attitude, though. They asked simple, straightforward questions about my sight, and I could answer them without being embarrassed. I feel that I now have a slightly different relationship with the children. If a child has misbehaved, and I have had to be really cross, when it's all over and I smile at the miscreant, just to show that there is no grudge, I can see from the way that child reacts whether or not a good relationship has been re-established. When I could not see at all, it was more difficult to be sure.

One evening, about this time, I received a phone call from Jenny De Yong, a freelance radio and television producer and director. She had read an article about me, she said, and would like to meet me. Jenny arrived on the train from London, complete with tape-recorder and dozens of tapes, one Thursday in September, just a few weeks after my first operation. She explained that she thought my story would make a good radio documentary, and outlined her plans to me.

At first, I didn't think about looking at Jenny, as she sat

beside me with the microphone. Because I didn't think of looking at the microphone, either, I forgot all about it, and found it very easy to relate my experiences of the past few months. Jenny told me afterwards that she found it quite strange at first, working so closely with someone who did not notice visual signals. Quite by chance, I looked round one day and was startled to realize that I could tell Jenny's response to the things I was saying by the expression on her face. We worked together for many hours, Jenny holding the microphone just inches away from me. I became fascinated by the silently changing expressions on her face as she made mental notes, no doubt of the value for her purposes of the things I was saying into her tape-recorder. During those sessions, I became very familiar with the tell-tale small puckerings of her brow, the quiet smile, her encouraging nod.

I was due to return to hospital in the middle of November for the second eye operation. The surgeon planned to do the second lens implant, and straighten the squint at the same time. Jenny had obtained permission to do some recording of my teaching, and to record various aspects of my stay in hospital, including the entire operation. The next time she came to Derbyshire she was accompanied by David, a quiet, unobtrusive sound engineer from the BBC. The sophisticated recording equipment he brought with him, however, was certainly anything but unobtrusive. It seemed to take up an enormous amount of space, poked and kicked you in various parts of your anatomy if you allowed it to get in your way, and its fur-wrapped microphone eavesdropped its way through the next ten days or so of my life with unswerving dedication.

Everything had been organized to the last little detail for the recording session at St Benedict's. Jenny and

David planned to sit in on my first lesson, so that they could get some idea of the sort of things I would be doing with the children. The second lesson, which would follow the same format, would be recorded. I was pleased that the recording was to be done in the morning. For one thing, the morning classes were more responsive than those I had in the afternoon, and as the day went on my voice began to show signs of strain, as I was doing a lot of work with noisy percussion instruments. The first lesson went really well, and the second was even better. The children were wonderfully co-operative. I couldn't have wished for a better performance if it had been scripted and rehearsed. I sighed with relief as the bell rang, indicating the end of morning lessons. Having dismissed the class, I became aware of Jenny and David muttering together in a far corner of the room.

'Everything OK?' I ventured.

'No, it's not.' Jenny's voice came as a note of doom. 'The recording equipment broke down during the first session,' she explained. 'That wasn't too serious, as we had a back-up set. Would you believe it? That broke down during the second session.'

All that effort, and they had nothing on tape. What on earth were they going to do? This was my last day at school before going into hospital. They decided that the only thing they could do would be to try to borrow equipment from Radio Derby, who rose magnificently to the occasion and very kindly lent them what they needed. We were all very grateful indeed. That afternoon the recording of the music lesson was successfully completed.

Totally exhausted, I arrived home to find that the furry eavesdropper had beaten me to it. I fed his voracious appetite for other people's business with the information that I was ready for a double whisky, dismissing Adam's complaint that there were lumps of something in the teapot with the suggestion that it was most probably a mouse. Helping me to dish up the meal, he managed to drop a rasher of bacon on the floor, and I ticked him off for wanting to put it on his plate. What a picture of a completely organized and harmonious home, all tucked away in that furry head, waiting to be regurgitated some time in the future for all who cared to listen.

One week later, and I was on my way back to hospital for the second operation. It was a wet, grey day. I looked at the line of rooftops across the road. Suddenly, I wanted so much to be able to see the tiles on the roofs. For some unaccountable reason, that seemed to be some sort of goal at which I must aim. As I looked at the raindrops on the car's windscreen, and the clear arc the wipers left, as they swept the little shiny drops away, I found myself remembering that, as a child, I had always minded the fact that I couldn't look out of the window and see the rain coming down. That had seemed important then, just as the tiles on the roofs seemed important now.

As we drove the nine miles to the hospital, my spirits felt as grey as the November day. I was anxious to avoid any publicity about my second operation. This was not secretiveness for its own sake, just that I felt very, very tired. I needed time and space, simply to breathe in and out, to be me, and to react however I needed to, to whatever the second operation might or might not bring about. I had to go ahead with the documentary, because that was a commitment I had undertaken, and I could count on Jenny to be sensitive. She knew how tired I was, and I knew her so well by now that her being there didn't seem to matter at all.

* * *

With my first eye operation, I had nothing to lose – or at least very little. I must have dared to hope, and had most certainly prayed, for some sort of successful outcome, but I had had no inkling of what to expect. After the removal of the dressings, I had been quite overwhelmed by the world that had gradually opened up before me. At first, until I learned to measure it by the yardstick of other people's sight, it seemed to me that no one needed to be able to see more than I could see. There was so much to look at that I didn't understand how anyone could possibly cope with more.

As the weeks passed, however, I came to realize the limitations of my estimated twenty to twenty-five per cent of normal vision, and looked forward with increasing impatience to the second operation. Without any grounds for doing so, I began to convince myself that it would give me twice as much sight as I already had. As with the first eye, there was no way of predicting the outcome of this second operation, and no one had implied that there was, but I began to conjure up an idea of 'twice as far', 'twice as clear', 'twice as detailed', and so on. It was all completely hypothetical, and outrageously fanciful, but absolutely real to me.

As soon as the bandages were removed that second time, I knew immediately that the operation had been worth while for, little by little, blurred objects assumed an identity. I could recognize the face of the nurse who had taken the dressings off, and could pick out the edge of the trolley beside her. I was disturbed, though, by a deep orange glow, as though I were looking through a dark amber glass. It was impossible for anyone to know, at such an early stage, what was causing this problem. It was possibly debris in the back of the eye and, if so, it would clear naturally in time. After a day or two it did clear, and there was a perceptible improvement in my vision – but I certainly didn't see twice as much. In time, it became obvious that the sight in the second eye was inferior to that in the first. Everything I saw with it was blurred, and lacked definition. That, however, mattered little when, from the very beginning, it became obvious that the operation had been very successful indeed cosmetically. The dreadful squint had gone, and my eyes moved together for the first time for many years.

A few days after it had gone away, the glaring orange glow returned. I could see things normally with the left eye, while at the same time, with the right, everything looked distorted and dark, and had almost a fluorescent appearance. At these times I became quite frustrated and tense. It was explained to me that sometimes, after an eye operation, a tiny blood-clot is present in the fluid at the back of the eye. As this moves about, it may, from time to time, float across the pupil, so that one is actually looking out through it – hence the dark glow. The clot would disperse in time. Once I understood, I coped more easily. Sometimes the glow disappears for days, sometimes it comes and goes several times in a day.

'If you could have a wish,' someone had asked me, 'what would you wish, regarding this second operation?' That was a challenge. Four months earlier, if I had known for certain that I would see the faces of my husband and my two sons, I would have said that I would never again wish for anything, for that would be all the world to me. And yet I heard myself saying now, 'If I had a wish, I would wish that I could see perfectly, just like you do, so that I could go anywhere, and do anything, whenever I wanted to, without having to listen and concentrate. If I could see like you do, I could go and live in the middle of a desert island if I wanted to. With sight like yours, even that would be easy.'

I'm sure that I would be terribly lonely on a desert

island and wouldn't enjoy it there at all, with or without perfect sight. On the other hand, not a single person had realized, until I pointed it out to them, how strongly the four conifers at the bottom of our garden resembled four old ladies in full, frilly skirts, with shawls pulled over their heads. Most of the time they just stand there, shoulder to shoulder, gazing out across the valley. But when the wind blows, it tosses and swirls their green skirts around them, and they lean towards each other like four old gossips, holding their shawls close around their nodding heads. Perhaps things like that are hidden from folk with normal eyes, for even when I have pointed it out, I haven't seen anyone give more than a cursory glance their way. Yet I could stand and watch them, nodding and gossiping in the wind, for half an hour or more.

In the centre of Belper there is a pub which serves morning coffee. I have called for years when out shopping. The atmosphere is friendly, and the landlord and patrons have raised enough money through the years to sponsor the training of five or six guide dogs. I have always sat in the same seat there. I was fascinated the first time I called in for coffee after my operation. I couldn't stop gazing at the plates that adorned the wall opposite the place where I had sat for years.

One morning I went to the ladies' room before going out to finish my shopping and I was reminded of going to the loo in the hospital, on the day the dressings were removed after my first operation. Then, stopping dead in my tracks, I thought consciously, 'Well, that is so ugly.' Bathroom fittings, too, struck me as being clumsy, and really unattractive. I hated looking at the plughole in the washbasin and bath, and the taps looked awkward, as though they were trying to pretend they were not really there at all. I shall never forget the first glimpse I had of myself in the mirror. I didn't like it – I really didn't like it at all. It was a real shock.

People had told me many times, through the years, that I am attractive and I liked to hear them say so; it boosted my self-confidence. I had only other people's word for it. Sometimes I wondered if they were saying it to be kind, and occasionally I egged people on to pay me compliments. That may sound conceited, but I think it was only using other people as though they were a mirror. I hadn't realized that, through the years, I had built up a clear visual picture of myself, based not on what I really looked like, but upon my ideal of attractiveness. The woman who looked back at me from the mirror bore no resemblance to that picture. The last time I had seen my hair it had been dark brown: this woman's hair was generously sprinkled with grey. I had been told many times, even by hairdressers, that my hair was attractive, too, but it didn't look attractive to me – I winced at the sight of it. Each time I stood before the mirror after that, I tried not to see the image that would not go away, the woman who turned her head when I turned mine, opened her mouth at exactly the moment I opened mine, who brushed her teeth, mockingly, the moment she saw me pick my toothbrush up. If I stole the quickest glance, there she was, glancing at me.

As I washed my hands that morning in the pub I looked up, expecting to see a frosted glass window – it had always seemed light in that corner. I jumped violently and let out quite a squeal. There, looking straight back at me, was another woman. I must be imagining it. To convince myself, I leaned towards what should have been a window. Imagine my horror when the woman on the other side of the washbasin leaned menacingly towards me. I put my hand to my mouth, thinking that I should faint if she came any nearer. I had obviously had the same effect upon her, for up went her hand to her mouth. Then the truth dawned on me. Above the washbasin was a mirror, and the light came in through a window to the right of it.

Another time, as I was wiping down the skirting-board in our bathroom, I caught sight of the most grotesque face I had ever seen. It was short and wide and squashed. I must be looking at something else that my brain couldn't interpret. No, there it was when I looked again, with its funny short, wide nose and its mouth half-open and distorted. Instinctively, I put my fingers out towards it. As they touched the shiny metal cover of the toilet-roll dispenser, I realized with relief that it was the distorted image of myself in the curved metal that had been grimacing at me so hideously. Now, I quite often make a face at myself in it, but make sure that the door is closed, so the family don't catch me amusing myself like that.

Since the second operation I sometimes suffer from double vision, particularly if I am tired. It doesn't bother me too much. If I get tired of watching two newsreaders on two television screens, I simply put my hand over one eye and all is normal once more.

One evening, though, as I washed my hands in the bathroom, I saw what looked like identical twins staring out at me from the large mirror over the washbasin. As I stared back at those two reflections of myself, my mind began to follow a strange train of thought. I began to wonder which of them was actually me. Which is the homely, domesticated one, I wondered, the one that takes a pride in folding the shirts so precisely, and hangs the washing just so on the line? It's probably the one on the left. In that case, the one on the right must be the confident one, who enjoys giving talks, and doesn't even look nervous in front of the television cameras. One of them would be dreadfully bored turning socks the right way out and sorting out the airing cupboard. On the other hand, one of them would go to pieces at the very thought of standing up in front of an audience and would be rendered quite speechless by the merest suggestion that she should actually talk to them. As I looked at them both, there in the mirror, their identical eyes, as they gazed back at me, did not betray in any way, which of the two faces really belonged to me.

This reminded me, as I pondered upon such an odd experience, how perturbed I had been, one night as a small child, wondering in which part of the body the real 'me' lived. It must surely be in my eyes, for it was with them that I saw the things that affected my life. But it was out of my mouth that my voice came, and said the things that came into my mind. In that case, perhaps I lived somewhere in the top of my head, or was it in that part of my chest that hurt so when the rough boys made fun of me or when Dad had to go away again at the end of his leave?

I smiled, and the two women in the mirror smiled their identical smiles back at me, and I felt that even if they knew the answer, they would keep it a secret between themselves.

CHAPTER 19

Bright Lights Everywhere

There had been interviews for Central TV's East Midlands Newsreel, during my first stay in hospital and soon after I had arrived home. But we were taken completely off balance by a phone call from London, two days after that, asking if we would all travel to the capital and appear next morning on TV-am. At first we refused the invitation. Such a journey would be far too tiring for me at this stage. It would all be very easy, we were told. A chauffeur-driven car would pick us up and take us to a hotel, where we would stay overnight. Next morning we would be driven to the studio and, after a short interview, the same car would bring us back home to Derbyshire. It certainly sounded very straightforward and it did seem rather silly to let such an opportunity slip by. After all, we argued, we would never have another opportunity to see inside a real television studio; and even if we were really awful in the interview, very few people who saw it would know us and those who did would have forgotten all about it within a week or two.

A couple of hours later, a large estate car drew up outside. In we piled, Ian, Ben, and myself – Adam was away at camp – and the two dogs jumped up into the back of the car. Off we set, on what, at any other time would have seemed an impossible and crazy adventure. Lennie, our driver, was so friendly and kind, we soon felt as though we had known him for ever. I must admit, though, that I felt like some kind of rustic. I didn't even really know what TV-am was, never having had time or inclination to watch television first thing in the morning.

As we travelled along the motorway, I was fascinated by a dark, horizontal line which seemed to lie across the road every now and again. As I watched it seemed to lift itself up slowly, so that I could see more and more sky between it and the ground. My focusing, at that time, was very slow indeed, so at first I was unaware of the sturdy pillars we passed as we went under the dark line, now way up above our heads. After a while I realized that these were roads, crossing the motorway. I told my companions what they looked like to me. When they actually thought about it, they understood what I meant about the dark lines which appeared to rise up out of the road. I had always disliked motorway journeys. The engine of the car took on such a monotonous note, and I would ask Ian at fairly frequent intervals if the road was very busy. On this occasion I didn't notice the note of the engine, and I actually enjoyed watching the traffic, trying to sort out whether the things that passed us were cars, lorries or vans.

Next morning, when we arrived at the studio at some unearthly hour, everyone was so helpful that I didn't suffer from stage-fright at all, although Ian and Ben told me afterwards that they had been very nervous. I suppose it was easier for me because, as the lights were very bright, I was unable to see the cameras with their operators and the friendly presenter appeared to me like just another person asking questions about my half-understood world of sight. I had put Victor's harness on him, so that people would know which was the working guide dog. Under the warm studio lights, it was not long before dear old Martin was fast asleep – I could hear his deep, relaxed breathing. When we watched the interview on video later we laughed, because whenever the dogs were mentioned, the camera zoomed in on Martin, sleeping away, and looking for all the world like an

enormous cream cushion with a black nose. I think
Victor, alert as usual, was hidden by a small table. I had
chosen a favourite red blouse to wear, and had to
congratulate myself on how perfectly it matched my poor
left eye, not yet recovered from the effects of the
operation. On our way home again, in Lennie's car, I
thought, That will be something to tell our grandchildren
about in the future.

I was astounded when, about a month later, Duncan
Wright, a researcher with TV-am, rang and asked if I
would like to visit Chorleywood College. I dimly remembered mentioning to someone at the studio that I would
love to see the place where I had spent most of my
teenage years. I had so often dreamed about the lovely
old house, particularly the great oak staircase that rose
from the beautiful entrance hall, which we used as a
common-room, to the landing above. I had slid down the
shiny banisters dozens of times, hoping to arrive at the
bottom before the gong stopped ringing for a meal. I had
always wished that I could show Ian the great old cedar
tree that had reputedly been planted at the time of the
great fire of London, and the alcove at the back of the
house, where I had been sitting that day when I really felt
that I had been called to the teaching profession. It was
thirty-three years since I had been there. Time, it is said,
allows us to remember only pleasant things, and my
memories of those seven years were all pleasant ones.

Duncan's investigations revealed that the girls had
moved to Worcester, to amalgamate with the college for
boys. The old house now stood almost empty, the last
remnants of furniture and equipment waiting to be taken
away. However, the RNIB very generously gave permission for us to visit my former school, although filming
would be restricted to the grounds around the house.
That was of little consequence to me. As the car moved

along the drive and rounded the sweep of the front lawn, I was certain that I must surely be dreaming about it all again. Stepping from the car, I was longing to cross the front lawn, to find out if the sundial was still there in the centre, surrounded by the rosebeds that used to give off such a sweet, gentle smell during the summer months. I was so excited that I completely forgot about the cameramen. Perhaps if I had thought about them, I would have toned down my excitement, just a little.

The RNIB had put Duncan in touch with Muriel Easter, herself blind, who had recently retired after teaching English at the school for many years. I had been taught by Muriel for a short time. As Ian and I rounded the corner of the winter garden, where sweet-smelling things had always grown, Muriel came out to meet us. Yes, I well remembered the gentle, quiet voice. She told me that her memories of me were that I had had a go at learning to make pillow lace. (The attempts, I thought privately, had been pretty abortive.) She remembered, too, my railings against the west wind, in my role as Dunois, in an open-air production of Shaw's *Saint Joan*. I hadn't thought about either of those things for years, but was pleased that those were the memories she had of me.

We looked at the old cedar tree, each of whose branches had had its own name. Some of the branches are missing, now, but I remembered the warm, rough texture of this erstwhile friend. Crossing to the alcove outside what had been the assembly hall and gym, I sat down on the garden seat there, absolutely certain that this was the self-same seat that had been there more than thirty years before. I felt as though we were suspended in some sort of fantastic time-capsule, that had hung in space while the rest of the world went rushing by. I am immensely grateful to TV-am and the RNIB for making this journey of nostalgia possible.

A week before Christmas, I was invited to appear on the programme again, to talk about my expectations and hopes for this first visual Christmas with my children. On arriving in the capital Joe, our driver, took us on a magnificent tour of London, showing us the Christmas lights and some of the more famous public places I had known for years, but not seen. That first, enchanting sight of London's Christmas lights will, I am sure, be a special memory for me for ever. During my wartime childhood there had been only the dimmest lights in the streets, and, although I had for some time been able to see the lights of the Christmas tree, street decorations had had no meaning for me at all. Now, as we drove along Regent Street, little Santas made all of lights were climbing up on rooftops made of lights, and going headfirst down chimney-pots made of lights. Once I had become used to the idea of it all, I could pick out the shapes of the roof-tops and windows, all made to look as though they were edged with snow. There in Trafalgar Square was the famous tree from Norway, looking very tall and straight and rather plain, but beautiful for all that. Pulling up opposite Harrods, I looked up at the front of the building, above the huge shop windows. The front wall seemed to be encrusted with thousands and thousands of little bulbs, strings and strings of lights, looking like beads that had been woven into a huge embroidery. I had seen designs made up of many tiny beads, on evening bags and things like that, only I had seen those with my fingers. Now, gradually, as I gazed at this enormous, lovely mass of intricately-woven lights, I could pick out what looked to me like the shape of simple Christmas trees.

On Joe drove, along the river, and the next time he stopped we were near St Paul's Cathedral. It was floodlit and, for some reason that I don't understand, I was able to see the building in a more detailed way than would have been possible in daylight. The shape of the dome stood out against the dark sky, and it appeared to be covered with a kind of tracery, rather like an elaborate iced cake. I could see what I thought must be a slender spire rising up from the middle of the dome. Imperfect though my sight of it must be, it was nevertheless breathtakingly lovely. Not for the first time, I had the strange feeling of seeing things that had been able to look at me for years. What an unexpectedly beautiful overture to a Christmas that was going to be packed full of delightful things to look at.

Christmas, always a special time, was particularly memorable that year. To the usual atmosphere of bustle, merriment, seasonal goodwill, was added a new and vibrant dimension – colour. Everything, everywhere, appeared to throb and pulsate with it, as though a giant heart-beat were pounding: brilliant reds and blues and greens in everything the eye lit upon. The drab greyness of winter, like my own old world of light and dark and shadows, had suddenly been replaced by a riot of sparkling, glittering beauty. As I stood, waiting for the lights to change at the busy crossing by the mill, I would often look across at the large old trees on the paved triangle where there are seats and telephone kiosks. Their leaves had fallen off while I was in hospital. I couldn't believe it when I first noticed their great dark, bare branches reaching up towards the wintry sky. One night just before Christmas, on my way back from town, as I waited in the dusk for the bleeps that would tell me it was safe to cross the busy road, I looked across as usual, and saw dozens of bright lights, twinkling among the branches, their bright colours shimmering as the breeze blew branches gently to and fro.

I loved the bright wrapping papers with their seasonal designs, and found it so much easier to pack the parcels now that I didn't have to keep checking with someone else whether or not I had the paper the right way round, with the pattern on the outside. When the cards began to arrive, I was touched by the fact that many of our friends had obviously chosen cards with bright, bold pictures, which were easy for me to see. As we decorated our own little tree, I was fascinated by the way the baubles caught the light from the window and the tiny coloured lights reflected their colour on to the wallpaper behind them. My Christmas world sizzled with warmth and brightness and beauty.

Ian brought some holly in one Sunday morning and asked if I could see the berries – he told me it was laden with them. I looked, but couldn't see anything. Instinctively I put my fingers out, and felt carefully amongst the stiff, prickly leaves. There they were – hard, smooth little berries, clustered together, nestling in knobbly, shiny heaps. Drawing my fingers away I looked again, and there they were, bright, shiny red, peeping out of the dark green shadows of the leaves. This is the way it is so often – my fingers seem to have to explain things to my brain before my eyes can understand what they are.

Suddenly, without warning, among all the festive fun, the tinsel, the lights and the nostalgic old tunes of Christmas, he was there, knock-knocking at the door, refusing to be left outside. I tried to ignore him, but he refused to go away. 'Who are you? What's it really all about?' he whispered through the crack in the door. 'Do you know, yet, which world you do belong to? Wasn't it easier before, really? It's a bit mind-blowing, isn't it, all this glitter? The brightness dazzles you. You are easily dazzled. I've seen you shading your eyes. I'm sure it really was easier before.' He was hissing through the letter-box now, determined to be heard. It was hard not to listen as his insistent voice whined on. That afternoon, a camera crew was coming to make a short piece of film. Someone had explained to me on the phone that every night during the week running up to Christmas they were going to round off the local newsreel with a happy story. I thought it a lovely idea, and agreed to allow mine to be one of them. Old bogey-man Kill-Joy had chosen that very day to have a go at me. Making a supreme effort to ignore him, I turned my attention to our decorations, the bright little tree, and the pile of presents in their colourful paper wrappings. By the time the men arrived with all their gear, the whispering had stopped and, tired of being ignored, the whisperer had shuffled off into the December shadows. And yet, when the piece went out on the air the following week, I fancied I saw his shadow flicker across the homely Christmas scene just for one second. I am sure I was the only one who saw it, though.

Our somewhat motley collection of family snaps and photographs has never really been sorted into any kind of order. From time to time one of the boys will light on a wallet of old snaps, while searching for something else, tucked away in a drawer. This gives rise to much merriment, usually at mine or Ian's expense. One evening during Christmas week, Adam produced one of these lost collections, and I wanted to know what he was laughing at. Having looked at it through my magnifying glass, I became fascinated; although my fascination was slightly tinged with horror at the pictures of a woman whom I did not recognize. Since she appeared with stubborn regularity with one or another of my children, or Ian, or family friends, sometimes accompanied by a dog, with or without a guide dog harness, I had no reason to doubt her to be myself. I became engrossed in this new experience of sharing fun and photographs with the family. Ian began to root about in one place after another, and Adam explained the less obvious pictures to me before passing them on to the others; we had a wonderful hour or so of reminiscing together. There were some lovely snaps of Adam, when he was three. It was strange actually to see him sitting on the little plastic motorbike I had carried out into the garden, and back indoors at bedtime, so often. Goodness, what an expanse of leg I was showing in the picture David had taken of me walking with Dana.

It was when we came to the head and shoulders of six-year-old Adam, with a shock of hair, sitting in front of some chequered wallpaper looking wise and solemn, that my eyes filled with tears; and when we got to the one where Ben, not yet two, had crawled into Adam's bed, and they both looked out, smiling roguishly at me as it seemed, the tears brimmed over and ran down my cheeks. Just for a few moments, then, I did mind not having seen them when they were small. The next moment, Adam had thrust another picture of me, with an unbelievably dreadful hairstyle, into my hand, and the tears gave way to shrieks of laughter once more.

It struck me, during those first months of discovery, how often it was quite mundane things that sent a pang of emotion coursing through my veins. One afternoon, I was drying an egg cup and, chancing to look down at it, I saw a little man with a smiling face and wearing a red coat and tall hat, painted on one side. Years before, Mum had given each of the boys an Easter egg in a pottery egg cup, and this must be one of them. As I continued to look at this small memento from the past, I felt my heart swelling up and up inside me, feeling as though it would burst out if it didn't stop swelling like that. I wanted, then, to look at other things that had meant so much to the boys during their baby days. As I searched upstairs for Big

Ted, and Jimmy Long-Legs, and Olly Owl, I was glad, probably for the first time ever, that my family are so loth to throw anything away.

On Christmas Eve, I spent a long time setting the table for dinner next day. This in itself was not unusual; on this occasion, though, it took ages. I kept stepping back to admire my handiwork. I had chosen a very dark green tablecloth. When I put the white lace place-mats on it, I was delighted with the strong contrast of the two colours: the delicate, lacy pattern showed up so well against the rich background. I was certain that I could see every detail. In my teens, I had often criticized my mother for having Sunday crockery and glasses, but now I am guilty of the same thing myself. As I took the best glasses from the cabinet and set them on the dark cloth, I was fascinated by the way in which they caught the light, and sparkled and twinkled, and looked as though they were shaking themselves all over, a little as a dog shakes as it comes out of water. I placed a green serviette into each glass, and stepped back again. Several times, during the day, I went back to have another look. It was very simple, not grand at all, but I loved to go and look at it.

I am not sure what I had expected of that first Christmas after my operations. Perhaps I had expected too much, not only of Christmas itself, but of myself, too. Understandably enough, a number of friends, said, 'You must be longing to see the boys' faces, when they open their presents.' And, indeed, that was so. I never ceased to be fascinated by their faces, even when they were engaged in the most ordinary occupations. I watched them as they read, and drew, or played with the dogs. I was fascinated by the way their expressions were changed by such emotions as anger, joy, or pity.

We have always opened our presents together, early in the morning, in our bedroom. I never felt at all excluded because I could not see what was happening at this time. I believed myself to be fully aware of their reactions and expressions, as they tore the paper off one gift, and then another. Quite automatically, they placed the contents of the parcels in my hands and explained how the different games or toys worked. I am quite sure that they have never even had to think about this – it is just something that they have always done. Nevertheless, after the opening ceremony, when they went off back to their own rooms, I was unable to think of anything else until every tiniest piece of discarded wrapping paper had been picked up and tidied away into a plastic bag.

The most outstanding memory for me, that morning, was this hitherto despised selection of torn and crumpled wrapping paper. As usual, the bed and floor were littered with it, but this time there was a difference. Before, it had been nothing more than useless, torn paper, which must be gathered up and got rid of before the dogs got hold of it and made even more mess. As I sat there then, however, clutching the bedclothes around me to keep warm, the bright little piles twinkled up at me from among the shadows of the covers, like bright, iridescent fish, swimming in a deep, dark pool. When I moved my feet under the covers, the fish jumped up out of the dark recesses and tumbled over each other, turning somersaults, bumping and jostling, and then lay exhausted for a while until, moving my feet again, I sent them all scattering off once more, bright and shining with the vibrant colours of Christmas Day.

In the afternoon, Ian called me into the kitchen. On the hillside, across the other side of the valley, shone a brilliant light. It flashed and sparkled like an enormous gem or a giant-sized star. Its light dazzled me, and I had to screw my eyes up. The sun, behind our house, was shining on a window at least a mile and a half away. I was fascinated and astonished, to think that I could see something which was so far away, and delighted that I had seen it shining like that on Christmas Day.

There had certainly been no shortage of glitter and glamour and colour during the festive season. I was very deeply touched by the determination of my family and friends that, this year, I should miss none of the wonderful things that there are to see when Christmas bursts, all dazzling light and laughter, into the gloom and grey of December. It had been a wonderful time, and I knew that I had been enormously privileged. No effort had been spared to enable me, with my adult mind yet strangely child-like, freshly-awakened eyes, to capture, and recapture, half-remembered, half-forgotten things, and others hitherto unknown. And yet, in spite of all that was new and exciting, the old way was not jostled out, did not take second place. The evocative sounds and smells of Christmas – the pealing of the church bells, drifting, now loud, now soft, on the lively breeze; the rich smell of the turkey, hissing gently in the oven; the pungent odour of candle-wax, when Ben blew the candle out after dinner – these held their place of time-tested honour among the green and gold and glitter that the new dimension of a little sight had added.

As, later that night, I stood as I so often do, looking out into the darkness of the night, my eyes drawn upwards to those countless sentinels upon the hills, I murmured a simple prayer of thanksgiving, out into the night. Sight and sound, warmth and love, had been inextricably woven together in the making of that lovely day. The gratitude I felt for each ached somewhere deep inside me, so I breathed it out into the chilly air and trusted the breeze to carry it where it should go.

CHAPTER 20

Seeing and Believing

A few days after Christmas another invitation for me to appear on TV-am found us touring London by car again, and this time the boys were with us. We were escorted by Sam Hall, a television news reporter, who spared no effort to ensure that we had a wonderfully memorable evening. I was just as enchanted by the sights and lights of London as I had been just a week before, but again it was St Paul's that made the greatest impact on me. There it stood, held close in the great arms of the dark night, magnificent with age and beauty.

What I felt and what I saw became inextricably intertwined. I couldn't tell whether it was the sight of the floodlit building, with the elegant shape of its dome and the stone tracery, or the awesome knowledge that that actual shape had stood there for centuries against the night sky of London; or was it that thirty years or so before I had stood beneath its shadow on many occasions without knowing what it was really like? It was almost as though the ancient dome had had some sort of advantage over me. I am not sure which of these thoughts and feelings and new experiences made some part of me, somewhere inside, feel as though it would swell up and burst with emotion. A sort of shaft went out from wherever I am, inside me, and touched the very top of the pinnacle, lighting the pathway from me to it with a silvery light, and saying 'I am here, and I have seen you. Tonight, my eyes have joined the countless others that have gazed with wonder upon your age and beauty and elegance. Perhaps I have not seen it all, as they see it, but what I have seen has made me hurt, it's so beautiful.'

And there, suddenly, further along the way, was Big Ben. Its big, round face shone out brightly, and I could see the enormous hands, which informed the world that the time was twenty-five minutes past seven. I really couldn't believe that I had actually seen, for myself, the time by Big Ben. Six months earlier, I could not even see the clock which had hung on my living-room wall for years, and had had to feel for it with my hands, whenever I wanted to dust it.

Increasingly, as the weeks went by, I became interested in television. Previously my attitude to television had been that I could take it or leave it, except for one or two programmes which I tried never to miss. I think I could see a vague flickering light from the set, although if the lamp near the set was on I could not distinguish one from the other. On the whole, I much preferred the radio, claiming that the programmes were of a much higher quality. I know that I would never have admitted that my comparative lack of enthusiasm for television was on account of my not being able to see it.

I was always surprised when people who did not know me well were disconcerted by my speaking of 'watching' the television. Since many blind people use visual language, this is not as extraordinary as it might seem. If I had enjoyed a programme with the family or friends, it would have been unnecessarily long-winded to explain, 'The family watched a wild-life programme, and I listened to it.' We all live in the same world, but some of us do some things a little differently. Wherever possible, in my opinion, we should try to use language which does not single us out. For instance, I would always say to the boys when they were small, 'Come here and let me see your hair is tidy.' This 'seeing', of course, was done with my fingers.

With my new ability to see with my eyes, the television became more and more meaningful to me, and sometimes I spent more time than I could spare watching it. I could not then, and still cannot, see small details, so that when there is a film or play with a lot of quick action or fine detail, I still have to ask what is happening. Nevertheless, I can see people's faces and clothes very clearly, and can follow with ease programmes where there is not too much going on at once. One night ice-skating was announced, and I was about to turn the set off when I became aware of figures gliding across the screen in a wonderfully graceful way. As I watched, they span and twirled and lifted their limbs into the most impossible-seeming positions, making lovely, elegant patterns there on the screen in front of me.

Another time a very young man was playing a piano concerto; I remember, most vividly, the strange feeling I had that I was intruding upon something very private. As the cameras went in very close on his face, I had the feeling that I had eavesdropped on someone's private confessions, which had been intended for God's ear alone. Another time, when listening rather than looking (as I often do simply because I often forget to look), I suddenly caught sight of a pianist who was wringing the heart out of a Brahms piano concerto. The music was wringing the heart out of me, too, it was so lovely. My eyes were moist with tears. And then, as I looked more closely, I wished I hadn't. There at the piano sat a very ordinary man, going a little bald. I went on watching, but something had gone from the music.

In January, at the beginning of term, I was thrilled to receive an invitation to augment the combined arts team at St Benedict's. Combined arts is usually a sort of mish-mash of music, art and drama, and I love teaching it more than anything else. I was pleased, too, that I would have a specific slot on the timetable, rather than just filling in for someone else. But the real reason for my delight stemmed from the fact that the school had sufficient confidence in my teaching abilities to give me a regular assignment for the rest of the school year, albeit only half a day each week.

Supply teaching is not easy for anyone, and for me there is the added difficulty of getting around quickly in strange and crowded buildings, sometimes having to cope with split sites. At St Benedict's there were two main teaching blocks separated by a five-minute walk up a long drive. This was complicated, at the time, by a fairly large building project. In places, the drive was pot-holed and very uneven, and lorries full of building materials were driving on and off the site for much of the time. There are also several temporary classrooms down a long, narrow path. Both Victor and I approached all this with far greater confidence after a trainer from the Leamington Spa centre had been to visit us. Members of staff, too, are always more than ready to offer help if they are available.

Most thrilling of all to me are the occasions when Victor and I are weaving our way between dozens of children at lesson changes and suddenly I feel a hand being slipped through my arm, and a child's voice asks, 'Do you want any help, Miss?' That is not, I think, an easy thing for a self-conscious teenager to do, especially nowadays. I believe that those children learn something of tremendous value from situations like this – something no textbook or ordinary teacher, however well-informed, could teach them. They have become involved in a real-life predicament and have coped with it, overcoming the natural reserve which seems to be a part of our make-up. Unfortunately, we still tend to preach integration and equality rather more than we practise it.

One morning I was asked to supervise a senior art class who were finishing off their examination work. As I stood at one end of the long art room, I suddenly became aware of a figure at the other end of the room. It looked like a girl with very fuzzy hair. She was extraordinarily still. A little later, I looked again and was surprised to see her still standing there. She wasn't being a nuisance or disturbing anyone; all the same, I felt I would soon have to say something, if only because she was wasting so much time. I didn't know the class, and waited for a few moments deciding on the best way to approach the girl. 'Do you intend to stand there for much longer?' would be a fair enough question in the circumstances but, to a senior class, would maybe sound somewhat autocratic and put their backs up. Just then another teacher came in.

'Who is that at the other end of the room?' I asked. 'She's been standing there ever since I came in.'

I knew this teacher well, fortunately, for, smiling, she informed me that the oh-so-still figure was a very large painting of Boy George.

One morning I awoke suddenly and wondered what on earth had startled me. Horrified, I became aware of the strong light that filled the room. We must have overslept. Strange that none of us had woken up. I could see my dressing-table, the photograph of Dana on the wall opposite the bed, the complete outline of the front and back windows. As I moved rapidly through the no-man's-land between sound sleep and complete wakefulness, I became aware that the light which illuminated the room, was like no light that I could remember. It was really rather eerie. Ian went on sleeping, quite oblivious to the fact that I was sitting bolt upright, turning my head this way and that, trying to ascertain the source of this strange light. A second glance towards the window did nothing to clarify the situation – indeed, it served only to deepen the mystery.

Craning my neck, I was astonished to see that the sky was still quite dark, but the road, through the front window, looked as bright and light as though the sun was shining. It hurt my eyes to look at it. As I looked, I became aware of dark, rectangular outlines, all filled in with the bright light. These, I realized, were the hedges and walls of the houses across the road, and the bright areas were the lawns and gardens. I looked up again towards the sky, and then the fact of the matter dawned upon me. The roofs of the houses opposite were bright and light, like the gardens and the road. It had snowed. How astounding, though, that the snow was so gleaming white that it lit up our bedroom, even though the sky was still dark. I could hardly wait for daylight.

Before I woke the boys, I looked, first out of the front and then the back windows. Already dark lines had appeared, to spoil the beautiful white ribbon of the road. The ugly dark lines zigzagged down the hill, spoiling the perfect whiteness I had seen in the night. Through the window at the back, however, I felt as though I were peeping through a crack in the side of the world into fairyland, or even heaven. The hillside looked like an enormous giant, who had humped himself under a pure white blanket. The trees and hedges criss-crossed all over it in sharp, dark lines. The houses, as I looked down on them, stood out darkly, too, but their roofs were pure white. For the first time I could easily see the chimneys sticking out, dark against the snowy roofs. And there it was, suddenly, the square, dark tower of the church, about a mile away, standing out as clear as a snow-scene on a Christmas card. Ever since my first operation, I had strained and strained my eyes, gazing and gazing into the higgledy-piggledy mass of houses on the hillside, trying to pick out St Peter's tower and the spire of the old Congregational church, but had always failed, and usually gave up, defeated and quite often frustrated.

As I looked at the tower, standing out so clearly in its snowy surroundings, I had a sense of tremendous personal achievement. Nonsensical as it may seem, when I am unable to see things that are apparently very easy to see, I almost invariably experience a sense of failure. When I am having what I call one of my 'bad seeing days', and make a silly mistake in front of other people – such as not being able to find my purchases on a shop counter, or reaching out towards the hinges instead of the handle of a door, I become thoroughly angry with myself, and cannot let the feeling of personal failure go out of my mind. I relive it a dozen times, and wonder how many people saw me doing such a silly thing. Probably none, usually.

There was no sense of failure on that first day of snow, in the spring of 1988. It was wonderful. Suddenly, something caught in my throat and snatched my heart up in its trembling hands. The conifers – my four old ladies – had decked themselves out in festive apparel to be a part of this sparkling white world. The green frills of their petticoats were trimmed with snowy lace, and as they bobbed and nodded their heads in the icy wind, I could see that they had put on matching white lacy caps. The silver birch and the eucalyptus shimmered and glistened with a new, almost ethereal light. For years I had hated the snow, thinking only how difficult it would be to get out with the dog, how filthy it would be everywhere, when it began to thaw, resenting its intrusion into the normal pattern of our lives. Now, with this wonderland of white beauty stretching out before me, merging at last into the whiteness of the sky, once again I felt a deep sense of gratitude for the unexpected gift of sight – even my kind of sight. I am certain that if I had perfect sight, my excitement, delight and amazement at what I saw that day could not have been greater.

More than a year of changing seasons had now revealed itself to my ever-hungry eyes. It was summer when the bit of sight that is all I have ever known, and so is everything to me, was re-awakened. My eyes could hardly tolerate light at all, and so I almost missed the luxuriant beauty of that most exotic of our seasons. I say 'almost', because the generosity of one of our local newspapers afforded me a treasured glimpse. This paper had featured me in an article just before my first operation, and my coming out of hospital coincided with its twenty-first birthday. To celebrate the happy outcome of the operation, I was taken with the whole family, including my mother and father, on a journey of nostalgia to some of the places in Derbyshire that I had long loved but never seen.

The first eye-opening surprise of the day was at Matlock. As we stood on the balcony of the cable-car centre, even my uninitiated eyes could not be unaware of the splendour of the surrounding countryside. The hillside plunged down so steeply that I felt as though the ground beneath my feet had turned an enormous somersault, and that my piece of firm earth might follow its example at any moment. I was awed as I looked down, down, down and saw the steep path winding out of sight, looking for all the world as though it were chasing after the tumbling ground. It looked as though there were great folds of grass and rock. I don't know why, but it reminded me of the feel of the top of a flaky pastry pie, with little blistered bits sticking up – if you touch them they collapse and cave in – all on an enormous scale.

Up in the cable car we hung motionless half-way across. Down below I saw two narrow ribbons, the road and the river. I couldn't see the railway. The river glistened, silvery in the sunlight. It was unspeakably exciting. I could actually see how far I was above the road – see it for myself, not just know because someone had described it to me. That was probably as important to me as if I had been able to see it in all its amazing glory.

During the rest of that magical day we visited other well-loved places, but afterwards, when I thought about it all, it was the trees in Chatsworth Park that had made the most lasting impression. They were, of course, in full leaf, but at that time I could not recognize colours, so I was unaware of their rich greenness. It was the elegance of their shapes, seen, I suppose, partly in silhouette that delighted me so much. The boughs hung full and heavy, seeming to dip around the upward curve of the trunk. The base of the trunk, as it curves outwards just before disappearing into the ground, had for me a special grace. The boughs dipped and swayed around it, giving the impression of full, swaying skirts. The reporter who covered the story, was too kind to say if she had been disappointed that I could only partially see all the lovely things they showed me. I most certainly was not. A partial view of such elegance and grandeur is a tremendously thrilling experience when for years it has been completely hidden away.

Since childhood, autumn has been the season I have most loved, with its smell of nutty brownness, its crisp mornings when cobwebs softly touch and cling to your cheeks. I loved to hear the leaves rustling as the wind blows them along in front of you as you walk. Blind people, even those who have never seen, can have a very deep appreciation of the beauties of nature. That first autumn, I was delighted to watch those rustling leaves as they scuttled along the road, looking for all the world as though they were running away from Victor and me as we walked down into town. As Victor looked after us both, watching where we were both going and leading me round obstacles, I was able to watch the scuttling, twisting leaves, fascinated by the capers they cut. I was aware of their different shades but, then, completely unable to see what colours they were.

My second sighted autumn, however, was magnificently colourful and brilliant. One morning, as I walked along the path under the trees that leads up to the church door, I was aware of an unusual brightness around my feet and, as I looked towards the edge of the path to get my bearings, I was astounded. Some attempt had been made to sweep the fallen leaves into piles, in case they became wet and slippery. As I looked, the oranges and yellows were so vivid, that I fancied I could hear them calling, 'We're here, we're here. You can see us, can't you?' I couldn't have missed them, they shone out like the dancing flames of a bonfire. 'O master craftsman,' I thought, with tears, not for the first time, brimming in my eyes, 'wherever thou art, how great thou art'. A day or two later, Ian brought three leaves in from the garden: one was green, one red, the third orange. The colours were so beautiful that, when I had finished looking, I could hardly bear to throw them away. And then I saw my first cobweb, ever, with the frost upon it, hanging between the outside light, by the back door, and the wall. It sparkled and glinted, and looked altogether too delicate and beautiful to be hanging there, in such a commonplace position. The phone rang and I had to stop looking; when I had time to go back, the next night, it had gone.

Spring was beautiful, of course, in its delicate way; but even though I could look at the fragile little snowdrops, and was enchanted by the cones of lilac hanging heavily on the trees at the bottom of the garden, it was the blackbird, trilling his jubilant morning chorus, and the heavy smell of broom that spoke most powerfully to me of spring. The added dimension of sight has, without doubt, served to enhance my already deep awareness of the beautiful things in this world, but the old way has not diminished in the smallest degree, and the evocative sounds and smells that set the memory alight continue to have a powerful impact.

Summer gained much, for me, for having colour added to its rich beauties. White clouds in a deep blue sky, the graceful trees, now resplendent in gowns of green. One night, when we were taking the dogs for a walk along a high, sandy track, I looked over a stone wall and saw the small fields, like a patchwork cover, criss-crossed by yet more stone walls. In the fields nearby, there were black and white cows, and one was walking with a tiny calf just behind it – a pretty sight. As I looked further across the valley, and raised my eyes towards the horizon, I felt sure my eyes must be playing tricks, for the landscape on that opposite hill shone out brightly in the evening light. As the sun had gone down, I couldn't understand where this brightness could be coming from. I was surprised, when Ian told me that those were fields of corn, that it really did look golden.

It seems strange that, since I have always sat huddled by the nearest source of heat on cold days, and shivered and grumbled at the very mention of frost, that I should have found the grey landscape of winter so especially moving. Whether out on foot or in the car, I was intrigued by the shapes of the naked trees, lifting bent and twisted arms towards the sky. For me, every one of them became endowed with almost human qualities.

And as nature revealed the contents of one treasure-chest after another, the treasure-chest of life did not fail to pull out from its store unexpected little trinkets that, in turn, delighted, surprised, and sometimes puzzled me.

CHAPTER 21

Special Appearances

I learned from Jenny De Yong that the programme she had made, based on my story, was to go out over the air during March, as one of a series of ten forty-five-minute documentaries, on Radio 4. My mind immediately went into a complete flurry, and I felt quite panic-stricken.

I couldn't understand my reaction. After all, during the hours we had spent together recording the material, I was fully aware what use was to be made of it. I had been tremendously interested in the project for its own sake, and in learning from Jenny how much work went into making a programme. Now the thought that not only I, but probably thousands of other people, were going to hear me – *me* – speaking out on Radio 4 filled me with alarm. I wondered if I had said anything, anything at all, the merest suggestion of something, that somebody would find offensive. It is so easy to do that without meaning to. I was fearful, too, that people might think me opinionated, or arrogant to presume that other people would want to hear about me. That had never occurred to me: Jenny had found my story interesting, and her enthusiasm had swept me along. In my anxiety I rang her a number of times for reassurance.

There would be two transmissions of the programme – one on Wednesday morning and a repeat the following Sunday evening. I think mine was the third in the series. On the Monday before the dreaded Wednesday the radio, as usual, was on at breakfast time. After the weather forecast, and just before the eight o'clock news, I was suddenly aware of my voice coming out of the speaker. I froze, horrified. During the next couple of days, I had a similar experience several times, and it never felt any better. I thought I had never heard so many trailers for a programme before, and just hoped that no one else recognized my voice.

On the Wednesday, I made a cup of coffee and was glad that the butcher had called earlier than usual: at least he wouldn't come in and catch me listening to myself. As I sat waiting, I couldn't have had worse stage-fright if I'd been sitting in Broadcasting House waiting to do it all live. Once the programme got under way, though, I forgot all about myself. Jenny had produced it so sensitively that I almost forgot it was about me. I was able to be quite objective about the whole thing, and at the end rang her up to congratulate her – to her relief: my anxiety had worried her.

A day or two after the documentary was broadcast, I received a phone call from Mary Clyne, a television producer at Pebble Mill in Birmingham. She told me that she had heard the documentary, and would like me to appear on a programme called 'Daytime Live' the following week.

Whenever this kind of invitation comes, my reaction is to pretend that I am not me. A large part of me secretly wants everything to be as it was before the dramatic turn of events in August 1987. On the other hand, I suspect that another part of me has lain dormant for years, ever since I was told that it would be impossible for me to pursue drama as a career. That part of me is intensely interested in every aspect of this hitherto unknown world into which I have been privileged to peep.

The two parts of my personality were once more in conflict. I desperately wanted to go to the studios at Pebble Mill – not because of being on television myself, but to savour its atmosphere, hear the technical talk of the cameramen, meet the researchers who gather together much of the material for the programmes, sit in the make-up room and then see on video afterwards the outcome of all the hard work and technical goings-on I didn't understand but found so exciting. So I agreed. Ian went with me and, as he drove along the dual carriageway, I was far more preoccupied with watching the backs of the enormous lorries on the road than with any thoughts of the ordeal ahead.

Just as at TV-am, there was such a relaxed, friendly atmosphere that I almost forgot the real purpose of being there. At least they knew about priorities, and offered us a cup of coffee straight away. At last I was sitting in my seat, with the cameras at the ready. I could hardly see anything in the bright, glaring lights of the studio. Suddenly I became aware of the studio audience: I had quite forgotten about that. I felt the world spinning around me – I wasn't sure whether I was sitting in the chair or twirling around in a kind of vacuum. Then, taking hold of the situation, I said to myself, 'Judy, you can't go whirling around in space like this, in front of the whole watching nation.' No sooner had I told myself that than Judy Spires was there, introducing me, and the interview had started. After that, I forgot all about nerves, the cameras, the live audience, and even the watching nation.

We arrived in Majorca two days after Easter Day, dismayed to see the low grey clouds and the rain coming down steadily, looking as though it had set in for days. Late in the afternoon, though, the clouds rolled away and the sun shone, and it continued to shine for the rest of the holiday. It was lovely to be there together, just the four of us. It was eighteen months since we'd had a holiday. Our summer holiday in Wales had been cancelled because of my eye operations.

One night, on our way back to the hotel after a walk into the town area, Ian stopped. The sky was very dark. He asked if I could see a star which was shining very brightly. I gazed up into the blackness and there it was, twinkling away. I had never seen a star before. That is my most precious memory of that holiday. Another experience I enjoyed was being able to watch for Ian, or Adam and Ben, if they had gone off to play pool and left me sitting in the hotel lounge. Because no one knew me there, I didn't feel self-conscious, and would put on my reading glasses and look at the pictures in some travel books we had taken with us. In the evenings, many of the guests played cards in the lounge. Childish as it may sound, I got a tremendous thrill from being able to play with cards that had no Braille symbols on them.

It was a lovely holiday, and on the flight home there was one more delightful experience for me. As we flew over the Pyrenees I could see the snow on top of the mountains. The clouds were white, like cotton wool, but there were breaks in the cloud and, looking down through them, I could make out great splashes of pure white. I was surprised that I could differentiate between the white of the clouds and the white of the snow. Once again, I became aware that what may seem like a very meagre amount of sight, to those who take their own for granted, can open up a whole new world of unknown wonders.

In the summer of 1987 a local businessman, Mr Andrew Winkler, retired. I had met him some years earlier, when he made a very generous donation to the Guide Dogs Association, and I had been asked to receive the cheque on the Association's behalf. I learned that Mr Winkler had raised a very large sum of money since then: moreover, he was going to augment that amount by adding to it any cheques he might receive on his retirement from a well-known local firm. Again, I was invited to receive the donation on behalf of the Guide Dogs Association. The cheque was to be presented during a champagne reception, and many local dignitaries were to be there, along with members of our local fund-raising branch of the Association, and Jean Vallance, then a training supervisor, came from the Leamington Spa training centre.

The cheque I received was for fifteen thousand pounds. In spite of this remarkably generous gesture, and the relative importance of the occasion and many of the other guests, Mr Winkler thanked me several times for having given up my time to attend the reception. I was impressed by his kindness and modesty. I thought I would probably never see him and his charming wife Audrey again, but I was wrong. Some time in May, the Princess Royal was to visit Derbyshire, and a lunch at which she would be the guest of honour had been arranged in the Co-op's Regency Rooms at Derby. Imagine my surprise when Mr Winkler telephoned to say that he and his wife were to be presented to the Princess at this luncheon, and then asked if Ian and I would like to go to it as their guests.

I was excited as I put on my new dress that morning, and hoped I looked as glamorous as I felt. Wendy, my social worker and good friend, had helped me choose my outfit, and I had been persuaded to be more adventurous than usual with my jewellery. The spring sunshine shone brightly. It was a perfect day for such an occasion. As we approached the Regency Rooms, the excited crowd was growing. There was a carnival atmosphere. I had been there a number of times in years gone by, but it looked much grander than I had imagined. The table at which we sat was very near the top table. As the Princess and her party came in, I quite unashamedly stared at her, turning right round to have as good a look as possible. It didn't seem quite the thing to do, and I could imagine, had my sons been there, that they would have expressed their disapproval of my behaviour. It did seem a pity, though, for the sake of my own dignity, to miss my first, and what might well be my last, close sight of a royal personage. We had a lovely time, it touched me to think that Mr and Mrs Winkler, who knew me only slightly, had been so imaginative in their expression of joy at my having regained some of my sight.

Some time that spring we received a communication from the office of the Lord Lieutenant of Derbyshire, informing us that our names had been submitted as possible guests at one of the royal garden parties which are held every summer at Buckingham Palace. I was astonished but, apart from telling my mother about it, I dismissed it from my mind, knowing that a choice had to be made from thousands of people, and believing there was no reason at all why we should be considered suitable. A few days after the Princess Royal's visit to Derbyshire, I picked up the letters (which usually fall on Victor, as his favourite spot is the red doormat just below the letterbox). One looked singularly imposing, and I couldn't wait until Ian came home from work to find out what it was. I fetched my magnifying glass and, peering at the stiff, white card, read 'The Lord Chamberlain is commanded, by Her Majesty the Queen, to invite Mr and Mrs Ian Taylor to a garden party at Buckingham Palace', etc. I read it again and again. I couldn't believe it was real.

It became a part of the strange feeling I have had again and again ever since I opened my eyes the morning after my first operation, that my life isn't real. At these times I feel as though my feet skim along a few inches above the ground, and the world goes on around me. I'm not a part of it, but I can't get out of it either. It's like a long, long dream, in which I can see, only I can't see properly, and the objects I look at get confused – I can see them but don't know what they are. People get confused, too, knowing that I can see because of the things I say, but not able to understand why I can't see as they do. Then, when I'm trying to explain it, my head feels as though every bit of it is drawing into a tight knot, right in the middle, and if it doesn't stop it will burst. I always expect, then, that I shall wake up. I almost do, but never quite. And then, in the next part of the dream, I meet a famous person, or appear on the television, or, as on that day, receive an invitation to a garden party at Buckingham Palace. How could such things happen to an ordinary person like me, unless I were dreaming?

After reading the card for about the fourth time, I phoned Ian at work. I don't think he thought it was a dream, but I'm sure he was as surprised and delighted and felt as honoured as I did. We never did discover who put our names forward, or why.

During the early weeks of summer, life settled into a quiet routine of domestic normality. I was teaching at least once a week – sometimes more. The weather was dry and Victor and I found the twenty-minute walk to the bus station, and a ride of similar duration on the bus, stimulating and relaxing in turn. I have not ceased to be surprised at how much I can see through the window of a bus. It really delights me when I am able to spot another vehicle nosing its way out of a side road or pedestrians on a crossing. The time passes quickly as I set myself challenges – how many landmarks can I recognize by sight? How many more this week than last? Perhaps it is partly because I am so relaxed that I appear to be able to see so many more things from the bus than when I am walking, partly because I am in an elevated position, with a panoramic view of the world around.

These were pleasant weeks. Two of my former colleagues from the secondary modern school in Belper were doing supply work. We sometimes went off at lunchtime, if we were only working for half a day, and had a leisurely lunch somewhere. On other occasions another friend, whose twins are the same age as Ben, and with whose family we have shared many a pleasant outing, would suggest a trip to one of the out-of-town supermarkets. That is quite a treat for me, I suppose because these places are usually only accessible by car, so they have a novelty value for people who, for one reason or another, are unable to drive.

At last the day of the garden party arrived. Jenny De Yong had invited us to go to her house for lunch and to change into our finery there. I had a new dress for the occasion, of course, rich, deep blue, with tiny cerise flowers here and there. One of the music teachers at school had been married at Easter, and she kindly offered to lend me the cerise silk hat and matching bag she had had for that occasion.

'What if it's windy, or wet, or both?' I asked, picturing the expensive hat somersaulting across soggy royal lawns, Ian, best-suited, in hot pursuit. Rachel insisted that she'd love to lend it to me, so I accepted, gratefully if a little fearfully. Wendy's loan of a frilly cerise umbrella helped to still my fears.

When we left Derby station, the morning was frowning and grey. As we came to the barrier at St Pancras, I looked back at the train, and had quite a shock: I wasn't expecting to see the sleek, modern lines of the diesel engine. I have travelled for years by train, and had always pictured a steam engine. Although I had always regretted the passing of the lovely rhythm of the steam train, I had given little if any thought to the appearance of its successor.

After lunch at Jenny's charming home overlooking the river in Chelsea she drove us to the Palace, insisting that we should go in through the big, main gate. Hundreds of people in smart new clothes were obviously bound for the same destination as us. As she drove, Jenny attempted to describe some of the outfits, particularly the hats. The rain had stopped, miraculously, it seemed, about an hour before, and the sun was shining brilliantly. Nevertheless, there was quite a strong breeze, so I had made sure the little pill-box hat was securely anchored with hairpins. As we stepped through the great gates of Buckingham Palace, I felt sure I must be dreaming. I was in such a state of excitement that the things I looked at weren't registering in my brain. As we passed through what I think must be reception rooms, I was aware of a great deal of deep red and gilt-work, and a lovely staircase. It was frustrating that my eyes would not focus more quickly, and had too little time to get used to the change of light. But I told myself that this was not a day to get frustrated about anything. It was a day when every moment must be enjoyed to the fullest.

Out in the garden, Ian left me sitting at a table and went off in search of tea. The snippets of conversation I heard, as I sat there, were fascinating. A band was playing, and the sky was very blue. I looked at the great windows of the Palace, and once again experienced that strange feeling of unreality. As a child I often dreamed that I had been invited to Buckingham Palace; now that it had come true, I was expecting any moment to be awakened by the alarm clock. We chatted to a number of pleasant people. The atmosphere was surprisingly relaxed, and very friendly. We actually did see a couple of hats going head-over-heels across the grass, but mine, thank goodness, remained firmly in place.

The mayor of somewhere-or-other, with whom we got into conversation and who had attended two previous garden parties, gave advice on how to ensure getting more than a fleeting glimpse of some of the royal personages who were present. It didn't seem quite right to go staring at people just because they were royal, but soon we noticed a large, orderly crowd gathering along one part of the lawn. We joined this crowd, rather shyly at first, at the very back. Ian is the very last person to push himself forward on any occasion, but suddenly he put a firm hand on either side of my waist, and gently eased me through gaps in the crowd, until I was in the very front row, next to an elderly lady in a wheelchair, who was on a visit from Australia.

Talking to someone in the crowd which faced us, I saw a rather small lady in a light-coloured outfit, with an enormous hat, and very high-heeled shoes. Ian whispered that it was the Queen Mother. I watched her as she moved along the line of people, stopping occasionally to talk to one person and another. Then she came across and bent down to the lady in the wheelchair, and for a few minutes they chatted, so easily you would have thought they knew each other. As she stood there, she was so close that I could have touched her, but I didn't need to indulge in an act which would have provoked the wrath of one of the gentlemen-at-arms who stood nearby: I could *see* the Queen Mother, with my own eyes.

Later, the Queen and Prince Philip walked by. My eyes had become accustomed to the strong summer light, by this time, and I saw, very clearly, the Queen's smile as she walked by, and the colour of her clothes and the umbrella she was carrying. The two hours went by so quickly. As we came out through a side gate and stood on the pavement outside, I half expected to look down and find that my blue dress had turned to dingy rags. I shall treasure the memory of that day for ever.

I had known about Anita for many years, although I only got to know her personally five or six years ago. She had lived next door to Ian when they were children, and for some time she had been the head of St Andrew's, a school for mentally handicapped children – referred to nowadays as children with severe learning difficulties. Anita invited me to spend a day at her school, and take the dog with me. As I went from one class to another, we talked to the children, in a way that they could understand, about Martin, and how he looked after me when I went out shopping or to visit friends. He was very gentle with the children, standing quietly and patiently, while they stroked him and investigated his lovely silky ears. One little chap, who was tiny for his age, followed us about for most of the day, and just couldn't keep his hands off the gentle giant of a dog, who must have seemed to him as large as a horse does to me. During the last session of the afternoon, I spent some time chatting with the sixteen- to eighteen-year-olds, who are referred to as 'further education students'. I was particularly struck by their friendliness, and by the expectation of the staff that they should make me, as a visitor, feel welcome, and take the responsibility of entertaining me, offering me biscuits, which they had made, and a cup of tea.

Anita mentioned that a blind girl was to join the school the next term, and that a full-time member of staff would be appointed to meet her special needs. I knew that I was one of the very small number of teachers in the county, at that time, qualified to teach visually handicapped children. I knew, too, that once I would have jumped at the challenge and applied for the post, leaving it until later to work out the practical considerations, supposing I should have been successful. That night, I told Ian about it, and he said that, when it was advertised, I should at least apply for the job. The more I thought about it, the more I convinced myself that I would be completely unsuitable for such work, and, as the school is quite inaccessible by public transport from where we live, I had a perfect excuse not to pursue the matter.

About this time I was given an opportunity to learn to use a piece of electronic equipment called an Optacon, which can enable blind people to read with the fingers from the printed page. I progressed well with the lessons, under the excellent tuition of Angela Neith, who was principally a mobility officer for the blind, but had also been trained to teach this particular technique to suitable blind people. The cost of the apparatus, at that time, was around four thousand pounds, so I knew that, for me, personal ownership was out of the question. A friend mentioned this to Lucy Orgill, a reporter on our local *Evening Telegraph*, and she came to see me during one of my twice-weekly lessons. The outcome was that she wrote an article about it, which, with a photograph, appeared in the paper. In the days that followed, Lucy received one or two anonymous donations from readers, which, they said, were to be used specifically to purchase this equipment for me. Then Trevor Coakley, a policeman who lives locally, came to see me. It appeared that he and some of his colleagues, had raised considerable sums of money in the past, and had used it to help disabled people and charitable causes in various ways. He told me that he had read the article in the *Evening Telegraph*, and would like to raise some money towards the cost of the equipment that I was learning to use. He mentioned, among other projects, a sponsored swim.

Not for the first time in my life, I was astonished and

moved by people's generosity. I was even more amazed when, a little while later, Anita wrote to tell me that she had shown the picture of me to some of the children in her school; they had expressed a wish to help and had undertaken several money-raising efforts on my behalf. Anita undertook to co-ordinate the whole project herself. I think it speaks well for the philosophy of the school that those who may often themselves be the recipients of charitable efforts, had been encouraged to look outwards and become involved in a scheme from which they would receive no personal benefit.

Altogether, the remarkable sum of just over a thousand pounds was reached. This was not, of course, enough to make possible the purchase of the original equipment for which it was intended, but after some research, and discussion with the main benefactors, Wendy contacted the Foundation for Communications for the Disabled. After Paul Hawes had demonstrated one or two items, I decided to spend the money on a lap-held word processor with a 'Mimmic' which will, when asked, read back what has been typed into the machine, letter by letter, or in single words or phrases or give orally any information for which it is asked. This wonder of technology has endless possibilities, and I hope I shall be able to use it in some way for the benefit of others.

I have to confess that I am not an apt pupil. The Foundation offers a wonderful service, and the patience of Paul and his assistant Mike, when they came to see me after I had had it for a few months and had made little progress, was almost embarrassing. I treat the 'voice' inside the machine with a distinct lack of deference and respect, and am inclined to give him a piece of my mind without the least attempt at tact or gentleness. Although Paul and Mike were very kind to me, I could hardly blame them if, after their two-hour session here, they went away distinctly of the opinion that I am better at making coffee than at operating computers and their like. Nevertheless I shall persevere, because I know that, once I have mastered it, this equipment, which could not have been mine but for the kindness and generosity of others, will be invaluable.

I had kept in touch through the years with Pam, probably my closest friend at St Gabriel's Teacher Training College. I was a bridesmaid at her wedding, and her husband David took all the photographs at ours. He teaches photography in a school of art in Salisbury. During the last few summers, with our families, we have visited each other's homes alternately. My boys particularly love David, who has a real gift for capturing the imagination of children of all ages. In 1988 it was our turn to visit Salisbury. For some reason my eyes were behaving badly during our visit, and the tiresome orange glow was there the whole time. It doesn't usually last so long. Nevertheless, there was plenty to look at, and I lost no opportunity to go sight-seeing.

I was enchanted by the beautiful cathedral, although I decided to concentrate on one very small area and sat for a long time gazing at the vaulted roof. I could not believe that, had I been able to touch those graceful arched folds above my head, my hands would have met with hard, unresponding stone. There was almost a liquid look about them – they seemed to flow, like the sea. The slender spire filled me with awe, partly because of its delicate shape, partly because of its height, and partly because of its age. I don't know any words that could adequately describe the way I felt as I looked at it, pointing straight up into the summer sky. I said that I would like to see it by night, floodlit, and we went out one evening especially for that purpose. We waited in an ancient pub beside the river for the light to fade. I don't know whether it was the quality of the liquid refreshment or the company and conversation that caused us to linger there too long but, just as we entered the cathedral close and lifted our eyes to behold its nocturnal splendour, the lights went off, leaving us in what seemed like pitch blackness.

During those five days, I was delighted by the animals in the Safari Park at Longleat. I had no idea that one had to look up quite so far to catch the eye of a giraffe, or that the stripes of a zebra were quite so starkly black and white. I was a little nonplussed by the camels' humps and, since the one I first saw was lying down, whatever grace it might possess was completely out of evidence. My companions all waited patiently until my eyes focused, in their slow way, so that I should miss none of the things they saw so automatically and with such unquestioning ease. They were determined I should not miss the tiger drinking from a puddle beside the road.

In the New Forest the patient ponies with their foals stood so still at the side of the road that I managed to see them without effort. I cannot remember ever having seen butterflies, and I was slightly dubious about going into the enormous glasshouses at the butterfly farm in the New Forest, but I am glad the family managed to persuade me. Adam was the soul of patience, finding beautiful specimens that looked as though they had settled for a while, and pointing with his hand close to them, so that I could follow the direction of his finger. I could not believe that there, before my eyes, were the real live shapes and colours that I had seen on birthday cards, and on many of the cards I had received upon leaving hospital. Visual experiences thronged in so thick and fast that there were times when I simply wanted to shut my eyes and switch off; but there were far too many good things to see, and I didn't intend to miss any of them.

I enjoyed poking around the gift shops with Pam. Anxious to demonstrate to her my ability to see some of their wares, I pointed out plates and tiles and other bric-à-brac displayed on the walls, far enough away for me to make them out clearly. But I spotted something I could not identify, something large and boldly striped. 'What's that?' I asked poor Pam, poking it with my index finger. She didn't need to answer. I felt the person who was wearing the stripy sweater stiffen under my prodding finger. Because she was so near to me, I hadn't seen the head which surmounted the eye-catching garment, or the legs which supported its wearer.

Just before the first anniversary of my operation, Duncan Wright of TV-am rang up and we had a general sort of conversation, mostly about holidays. Somehow we got on to the subject of television, and I told him how much I had enjoyed watching the ice-skating, adding that I would be interested to see a ballet some time. A few days later I was invited to appear on the programme once again, to talk about some of the experiences of the past year. As Ian was unable to have time off work, Joy, a friend of many years' standing, was happy to go to London with me and, at the request of the producer I imagine, Victor went along too. It was getting late when we arrived, but I was anxious for Victor to have a good run before we checked in at the hotel, so our friendly driver took us to Regent's Park. It was a lovely summer evening, and the trees gave off a warm, green smell, as we walked beneath them. Looking up into their dark greenness, I thought they had a heavy-laden look. Our driver had taken us to a point from which we had a very clear view of the mosque with its exotic golden roof.

After the usual early morning call, Joy took Victor to a nearby park, while I finished getting ready. On her return, she reported that Victor had thoroughly enjoyed his run, the Duchess of York had given birth to a little girl, and that she had seen a car outside which seemed to be the one that would take us to the studio. The driver, she told me, had smiled at Victor in a very friendly way. When I emerged from the hotel, the driver and I both smiled as he planted a friendly kiss on my cheek. It was Len, who had driven us from Belper almost exactly a year before, and for whom I had cherished a feeling of special affection ever since that first astonishing visit to a television studio.

At the studio, of course, the subject on everybody's lips was the new daughter of the Duke and Duchess of York, but they managed to find a space to interview me and there were a couple of lovely close-up shots of Victor. Richard Keyes, one of the presenters, remarked that he understood that one of my ambitions, now that I had some sight, was to see a live performance of a ballet. He said that they had tried to get tickets for me to see the opening night of the Kirov Ballet at the Royal Opera House, Covent Garden; that had not been possible, but he gave me tickets for that morning's final full dress rehearsal, at which the press and a specially invited audience would be present. I was completely astounded, and delighted too.

As we sat in our box, waiting for the performance to begin, I had plenty of time to look around at the beautiful auditorium. As my eyes slowly became accustomed to the light, I could see the ornate decorative work, picked out in gilt, shining softly in the dimness. There were wall lights with deep red shades. Most of all, I was attracted by the curved sweep of balustrade at the front of each level, rising up and up almost to the ceiling. I knew nothing of the story, or the music, of *Le Corsaire*, the ballet we were about to see, but it didn't matter. The atmosphere was charged with anticipation of something special. Nor did it matter that I could not see the faces of the dancers: I couldn't even tell whether they were men or women, except by their clothes. I could see the beautiful groups they formed, as they moved around the stage, and their many-coloured costumes.

It was in the second act, when the dancers wore the traditional tutus, like the ballet dancers on top of musical boxes, that I could see them best, and easily distinguish between the male and female dancers. The figures of the women, in particular, showed up against the comparatively dark backdrop, and I could see their long, graceful limbs as they stepped this way and that, lifting their arms, bending their bodies like white birds engaged in some mysterious ritual. And then came what I suppose was a pas de deux. As the ballet dancer lifted his partner high into the air, and she stretched her limbs into a pose of complete elegance and grace, my breath caught in my throat and I felt tears prickling in my eyes. I don't know why it affected me so. I wonder how I would have reacted to my first ballet if I had been able to see it properly, as the rest of the audience saw it? Again I had that strange feeling that this was not happening to me.

I had been happy to leave Victor with Len, confident that Len would look after him well, and they had had a lovely walk in the sunshine, beside the Serpentine. Len had a message, received over his car radio, for me to phone the TV-am studios. By the time I got through, I was beginning to feel quite unwell, and was very dubious about the request that I should stay another night in London and appear on the next day's programme. (It turned out that I had some sort of virus infection, which left me feeling very low for about two weeks.) I knew, too, that it would be very difficult to get hold of Ian, to make arrangements for the boys. Eventually we reached a compromise: I agreed to go direct from home to the studio in Birmingham next morning.

It takes about an hour and a quarter to drive from our house to Birmingham – longer if the roads are busy, of course. As my slot was scheduled for eight-fifteen, a taxi was to pick me up at six-thirty. At seven o'clock it had not arrived: it had broken down, I was told, and another was on its way. A brand new, London-type taxi drew up fifteen minutes later and rushed me and Victor through increasingly dense traffic, with voices checking on our whereabouts at intervals over the driver's radio. When we got into Birmingham traffic conditions were appalling; by now I was convinced that it was a wasted journey, but I kept my thoughts to myself. As we came to a halt outside the television studios, the door was opened and firm hands grasped my arm. I hardly remember covering the distance from the taxi to the sofa, on which I suddenly became aware that I was sitting, Victor by my feet. I heard someone whisper 'You're on in ninety seconds', and felt something being inserted into my ear and a microphone being clipped into place. Luckily, while I had been waiting at home for the late car, I had put my make-up on except for the lipstick, and that I had applied in one of the traffic jams in Birmingham. Suddenly I heard the voice of one of the London presenters in my left ear, and realized that the interview had begun. It didn't go at all badly – I didn't have time to think about nerves.

After the interview, and a more than welcome cup of coffee, Victor and I climbed into another large taxi and travelled, at a rather more leisurely pace, back to Derbyshire. I had to do some shopping, so went straight into Belper without bothering to change my dress. As we shopped, Victor and I were greeted by several people, who said to us with some amazement, 'It's less than two hours since I saw you two on the telly.' As it turned out, a second night in London would have been far simpler, but on reflection, I really rather enjoyed all the excitement, and it will be a good tale to tell my grandchildren some day.

CHAPTER 22

Illuminations

September. Beautiful September, the herald of volup-
tuous, golden autumn – the season I loved most. The
trees still wore their summer green, but this year, as they
exchanged it for the brighter hues they put on before
going into winter mourning, I would be able to see and
recognize the brilliant autumnal tints.

Adam was going into the sixth form at his school, and
Ben was starting at Belper school. For two years he would
be at the school where I had taught for thirteen years. Just
before the end of the summer term, Anita had asked if I
would be interested in taking some music classes at St
Andrew's School once a week. I agreed to give it a try, but
privately felt very doubtful of my ability to cope with
'those sort of children'. Anyway, the six week's summer
holiday was upon us, and there was no need to think
about it for the time being. Now my first day at St
Andrew's was approaching fast. I gave a great deal of
thought to the sorts of things I might do there. Although I
knew that I was dreadfully nervous about this new
venture, and would probably make numerous mistakes,
of one thing I was quite certain. Whatever I did with the
children, it must be worth while, and I must do it to the
very best of my ability.

From the moment I set foot inside the school, that first
Wednesday morning, I was struck by the warm friendliness of both staff and students. I was let down very
lightly at first, spending some time in each class just
getting to know the children. It soon became obvious that
the staff had a very straightforward, 'normal' approach

to their pupils, however severely handicapped they might be. There was nothing patronizing in their attitude. Each child was treated with the respect to which, I believe, all human beings are entitled, but which they are often denied by a society which, largely through no fault of its own, lacks understanding. At first I found it difficult to get around in the rather complicated building, and tried hard not to be alarmed, and not too doubtful that I should get there, when one of the pupils was asked to show me the way back to the staff room. I quickly learned better, and soon looked forward to chatting with Kevin and Anne and Wain and Nicky, to mention but a few of them, as we made our way along the corridors, often followed by a small retinue of pupils who had been made responsible for putting the instruments away.

When I am with the children, I tend to think of them as being neither handicapped nor not handicapped. They are just themselves. Emily has a lovely face and lots of courage, Earl has a wonderful smile. Jonathan is enthusiastic about everything he does, and Brian makes the most enormous effort, in his quiet way, to get things right. They are simply children, and they could so easily have been mine. Within the first few weeks I developed a warm affection for them, and, contrary to all my expectations, began to look forward to being with them each Wednesday. I am sure that I must make many mistakes, but both staff and pupils have been wonderfully patient with any blunders I may unwittingly have made, and greet me each week as though they are glad to see me again.

Some of the children are unable to communicate through normal language, and some have hearing problems. For this reason, the staff learn to 'sign'. I am told that this method of communication can be very beautiful to watch, and that it can be wonderfully expressive. On several Wednesdays, a number of the staff stayed for an hour to learn signing. As I had to wait, in any case, for my lift home, I asked if I might join the class. We were divided into pairs. One partner sat with his or her back to a picture on the wall, and the other one's assignment was to describe it as fully as possible, using only signs. I am not able to see the sometimes quick, small movements of my partner's hands, unless she is wearing a dark dress to make a contrasting background for her hands. I had the task, therefore, of describing, without using any words, a house with a television aerial and open windows, with curtains fluttering in the breeze. The doors of an attached garage were open, showing a car inside. In the garden, a woman with a shopping-bag was walking past a duck and a pig and, just for good measure, an aeroplane had landed on the front lawn.

This would have been a somewhat formidable task for someone used to living in a predominantly visual world. Can you imagine the difficulties of one who had spent the major part of her life in a world where sound is of paramount importance, and much of the information she has needed has been gained through its correct interpretation? In fact, my partner and I were doing quite well until we came to the pig. I thought I had displayed considerable ingenuity as, pinching my nose with one hand, I attempted to describe the shape of a curly tail with the other; in case she should be a little slow on the uptake, I mouthed 'phew', at the same time. After that, no one ever took my attempts to learn 'Mackerton', quite seriously, but they kindly allowed me to continue to join them in the class.

Also during that September, Tony Nicholson came to see me. He explained that the school at which he was teaching, in Derby – a smallish comprehensive – was due to close in July. In 1903 the school had raised money for a sledge dog for one of Scott's Antarctic expeditions. The staff and pupils had decided that it would be good to raise a thousand pounds to sponsor a guide dog in the last year of the school's life. He asked if I would go, with Victor, to talk to the school in an assembly. For the first time ever, after a talk, I was asked to stay for the rest of the day, and put on my other hat and take classes, as a supply teacher was needed. The talk had broken much ice, and the children soon put into practice some of the things I had told them in the assembly about helping people with poor or no sight. In the very complicated school building, I was never short of a pair of helping hands. I was delighted when, at the end of the school day, the deputy head asked if I would go again at the end of the week. It delighted me, too, when a couple of children arrived at the staffroom door to enquire if I would like some assistance in getting to my next lesson. I overheard one of the male teachers commenting to another, 'That's the sort of thing no textbook can teach them.' Victor and I became familiar figures on the awkward staircases there. One day I overheard a first-year child say, 'Oh good, Victor's going to teach us today.' Perhaps that's not as funny as it sounds. I am sure that these children will have learnt, in a truly practical way, something that they will remember long after classroom days are done.

We had first got to know Wales through Pat, one of the group from St Peter's who had volunteered to look after Ben, when he was small, while I went out shopping with Martin. She often talked of happy family holidays spent at Mr and Mrs Owen's farm, the little village of Tudweiliog nearby, the grandeur of Snowdonia visible from the sitting-room window, trips to slate mines and rides on the Blaenau-Ffestiniog steam railway. It sounded the sort of holiday we would enjoy, and when she asked us to join them there one summer we were delighted to accept. Pat and John's son is just a little older than Adam, and their daughter comes somewhere between Adam and Ben.

The moment I set foot inside the farmhouse, at Towen on the Llyn Peninsula, I knew it was special. The front door opens into the kitchen, which felt very cool but smelt fresh and clean. Someone thought to point out to me immediately the sharp edge of a cupboard, directly above the table, the sort of thing that tends to imprint itself indelibly on a blind person's mind. Failure to remember such seemingly trivial details can result in a very painful crack on the head or face if, for instance, you hear a child call out suddenly, and jump up quickly to avert, or rescue him from, some disaster. The geography of the sink, too, with its tap far higher up than normal, was pointed out to me. The comfortable sitting-room, with its solid old table and dresser (and armchairs which never stayed in the same place for long, so making an ever-changing obstacle course), felt homely and lived-in. Upstairs, the comfortable bedrooms evoked immediate memories of my childhood. There was that very same smell that had been so much a part of my parents' home, something I had associated with first coming home each holiday from boarding school.

As I stood in the warm, roomy bathroom, I heard the clanking of an iron gate and feet scraping across gravel. Someone knocked at a door below the bathroom window, but when I heard the door open and unfamiliar voices talking, I knew it was nothing to do with us. Later, when we had unpacked and had a cup of tea, we went out, across the farmyard, and on to a lane, where our own feet made the scrunching noise I had heard earlier. Next we stopped, while the clanking iron gate was opened, and then shut, behind us. We followed a track across a field: I knew it was narrow, because if I put my foot slightly too far to the left or right, I was walking with one foot several inches higher than the other, probably demonstrating the gait of the drunken sailor in the song. As we crossed the small field, I could hear children's voices, and the bleating of sheep.

Suddenly we turned a corner, the path beneath my feet became very rough, and a cool breeze seemed to slap me gently but firmly on the cheek. In that instant, the sounds made by the children and the sheep were silenced, with dramatic suddenness, and replaced by the evocative sound of the incoming waves of the sea. We stood there for a moment, high up on the rocky path, breathing in the sea-laden air, listening to the swish and rumble and boom and roar of the waves, as they broke upon the sand and lashed around the rocks. 'Oh Judy,' Pat said, almost embarrassed, I could tell, by the strength of her own feeling. 'It is so beautiful here. I would love you to be able to see the sun set over the sea.'

As we went on down the steep, rocky path, half natural, half man-made, and my feet sank at the bottom of it into the fine, warm sand, I thought to myself that I didn't need to see it, for the beauty had already conveyed itself to me, by the sounds I heard, the feel of changing surfaces beneath my feet, the smell of sea and country-side on the gentle breeze, and the aura of peace and tranquillity that inhabits the place, no matter how many holidaymakers may rest or play in the little bay among the rocks.

That was a wonderful week. The sun shone every day. The children loved the farm dogs, the goat, the pig, who seemed to be treated almost like a dog, and the ducks on the farmyard pond. The holiday ended all too quickly, but we all knew, for certain, that we would go there again. And that was exactly what we did – for seven consecutive years. We had planned an eighth year at Towen, but that was not to be. The life-changing meeting with Mr Salem, the operation and all that was to follow, intervened.

Within the annual pilgrimage to Wales there were mini-pilgrimages – places we must visit every time, for one reason or another; places that meant something special to one of us, or all of us. I suppose, though, for the children, the beach was where they most liked to be. When they were little I joined in the fun of the beach with them, making sandcastles and sometimes paddling at the edge of the sea. As they grew older and bigger, the games became more boisterous until, at last, beach football, cricket and tennis took over from sandcastles, and left me more or less redundant. Sometimes we womenfolk would go off in the car to a nearby town, or to a little café further along the peninsula. But I must have spent many hours, over the years, more or less alone on the beach, listening to music through headphones, knitting, or even reading books in Braille – although that always makes me feel rather conspicuous, because of their enormous size.

I didn't mind being on my own. Over the years, I have managed to teach myself to keep boredom at bay. But if I am really honest, there have been times when, listening to all the noise and fun of the beach, I have felt sad that I could not join in with the ball-games that our children were enjoying. I have to admit, too, that there are times when the inability to do so has left me feeling somewhat inadequate. But these kinds of negative thoughts produce nothing worthwhile, so I have more or less developed a technique of switching them off; I hope I haven't voiced them very often, or that others will forgive me for the occasions when I have.

The last Monday in September is always a holiday for
Ian, in lieu of the August Bank Holiday Monday. I was
really surprised when, one day, he told me that he had
been wondering about going off to Tudweiliog for the
day, so that I could see the mountains with heather on
them, and Towen bay, before it became too wintry. I had
looked at a photograph that a friend had taken of it from
the little rocky path, but I couldn't work it all out. It didn't
seem to bear any resemblance at all to the way that I had
pictured it. I had always imagined it golden, and blue,
and green.

Everyone thought us quite crazy, making the four-
hour journey each way in a day. I was very excited, and
longed for the day to arrive. When it came it was not one
of my good seeing days, but I didn't even really care
about that. The journey went well, and it seemed no time
before we had crossed the border into Wales. And then,
suddenly, there they were – the mountains I had so often
heard described now appeared before my eyes, looking
like great puddings that had just been turned upside-
down out of enormous basins. They rolled on, one after
another, on as far as I could see, sometimes to the right,
then to the left, and others directly in front of us, it
seemed. Although I couldn't see what it was, I was able
to distinguish a kind of rough texture all over them. At
the top was a definite, dark, purplish line, and then the
sky. It looked for all the world, I thought as we drove
along, as though some gigantic hand had gathered them
up at the top, squeezed the edges together, and folded
them over, like an enormous pasty, so that the
mountains would not spill over untidily into the sky, or
the clouds fall down inside the mountain-tops, and get
lost there in the mysterious interior of the mountainside.

We stopped, and got out of the car. Just beyond my
feet, the ground seemed to disappear and, looking to see

where it had gone, my eyes could follow the grass and rustling bracken down, down, down, like an upside-down mountain, stretching away, further than I could see, without a neat margin, like that of the mountain-tops up in the sky. We picked a bunch of the lovely purple heather, and got back into the car. I felt sad when at last we left the mountains, with their dark-hemmed tops, behind.

Ian drove the car into the farmyard, and switched off the engine. 'There's Mrs Owen,' he said.

'Ian, I don't want to see her,' I told him, sheer panic rising inside me. All the way along the lane to the farm, a strange tight feeling had spread from the pit of my stomach, right up into my throat. To me, the Owens had been warm, kindly people, with lilting Welsh voices. I wasn't quite sure that I wanted them to have faces. I supposed I had endowed this place with half-mythical qualities, and I wanted them to go on being a part of the myth. The next moment I could be in no doubt that the dark-haired woman with the bright, smiling face was the owner of the soft, sing-song voice I had known for so long. She was astonished and, I am sure, delighted to see us. I felt unaccountably shy as I looked back at the eyes that were looking at me.

The farmyard was an absolute delight, just like a farmyard in a picture book, with hens and cockerels strutting and scratching about. I have always been absolutely terrified of birds. Suddenly I realized that these were very close to me indeed, and that I hadn't panicked at all. My preoccupation with watching them bobbing and curtsying there, had completely taken precedence over my customary fear. A little black and white sheepdog came running up, and sat close to my legs, as I stroked her smooth head. I could hear pigs grunting in the sty across the yard, but couldn't see them

from where we stood. The house looked tall and angular,
and very grey.

Leaving the car in the farmyard, Ian and I crossed the
lane and opened the clanking gate into the field that leads
across to the headland and the rocky path down to the
bay. I could see the narrow grey track as it ran ahead of
me, the tufted grass on either side looking as though it
had stepped back a pace to allow the path to scamper by.
As we reached the point at which the path becomes
rougher and turns, we turned, too, and there it was – the
breeze on my cheek, the sound of waves in my ears.

Ian told me to look ahead, as far as I could see, down
the rocky path. There, far below my feet, I could see a
golden triangle, nestling among what looked like black
hills. I knew that the golden triangle must be sand, but
couldn't understand why the hills were so black, or why
they formed a triangle. And then, how could that triangle
of gold really be the beach – all of it? It had felt quite large
when we had walked across it to make our 'camp' on the
further side. I had always thought of it as being semi-
circular, too, with gentle grassy slopes rising to the fields
where the sheep grazed above.

As we walked down the steep path, I understood for
the first time why my mother, the year she came, had
cautioned me so often to stay close to her as we
clambered down. A jagged wall of rocks sloped steeply
down to the sand and sea, far, far below. How strange. I
had never imagined any danger there. As we climbed on
down, the beach opened up to the right, and I could see
the water, glinting in the pale autumn light. The bay was
deserted. There were the prints of a horse's hoofs, but
civilization might have been a thousand miles away. I
stood there spellbound, stunned by the majestic
grandeur all around. Surely this wasn't the place where I
had sat and listened to my cassettes, and knitted, and

had picnics and barbecues. Here was a wild, ancient sort of beauty, that knew nothing of sandcastles and buckets and spades.

Standing among those dark, ancient rocks, I felt tiny and insignificant, and yet strangely a part of its aura of timelessness. It was almost frighteningly beautiful. I thought that if ever I met God face to face, it would be in a place like this. We wandered down to the edge of the sea. There was a lonely rock, much smaller than the others, around which the waves lapped, slapping it and then receding playfully, before it had a chance to slap them back. It reminded me of the boys who used to taunt little Specky Four-eyes, and run off too quickly for her to catch up with them. I saw the sky reflected in pools which had formed in rough hollow bowls among the rocks. Ian told me that there were tiny fish swimming in them, dozens of them, but I couldn't see those. It didn't matter. I had seen waves, some large, some no more than ripples, breaking around the foot of a lonely rock, pools in which the sky could see its cloudy face, and dark rocks as old and venerable as time.

Although I had known that this place would be beautiful, there was a magnificence here far greater than anything I had expected, and which I found almost impossible to take in. I wanted time to stand still, to allow me to sort it all out, in my slow way, so that it became a part of my understanding. I couldn't believe that what had always been just a well-loved family holiday beach could have affected me, at first sight, so deeply, so profoundly, somewhere inside where it ached.

'How did your holiday in Majorca go? Did you have a wonderful time?' It was Mary Clyne from Pebble Mill, phoning to say that some of the guests who had appeared on 'Daytime Live' in the last series were to be invited back to the studio, and I was one of those to be asked. I told her that we had had a really good holiday at Easter. 'Were there lots of exciting things to see?' was her next question. To which I replied that the sea had been beautiful, and the palm trees had fascinated me and so had the mountains. Following that train of thought, I went on, 'But nothing there amazed me nearly as much as the places we saw in North Wales, one day last week. I hadn't imagined it to be nearly so beautiful.' I heard a sharp intake of breath, down the telephone wire. 'Would you talk about that on the programme?' Mary asked.

Two appearances followed – one the following Monday, and a second on the Tuesday of the following week. That was a beautiful autumn day and, as I got out of the car at the studio, the vibrant colours of the leaves that blew around my feet delighted me yet again. As it was the school half-term holiday, Ben had gone with me. I don't remember who I was chatting to when I became aware of a strangely familiar voice, greeting Ben with great warmth and friendliness. Where on earth had I heard that voice? It belonged somewhere in the past.

As I pondered, someone introduced me to Floella Benjamin, one of the presenters for that day. Little wonder I recognized her voice: Floella had seemed almost like one of the family some years before. She had been part of the 'rescue kit' when, towards the end of a long day with a toddler, when I was running out of resources and, more important, energy, there she was at the touch of a switch, with Big and Little Ted, Jemima and Hamble, all energy and laughter and fun. For twenty blessed minutes or so, I could just sit back and let 'Play School' take over, while I got up enough steam to go and start preparing the evening meal.

In answer to the question, 'Are there any places or things that you would still like to see?' and thinking of how I had been delighted by the illuminated, decorated boats at Matlock Bath, at the end of the summer, I said that I would love to see the illuminations at Blackpool some day. I was amazed to be told that 'Daytime Live' intended to do just that – to take me, with my family, to spend a weekend at Blackpool to see the famous illuminations there. Seaside holidays were out of the question during my wartime childhood. I suppose that, by the time holiday-makers were once again free to stay at coastal resorts, I must have been twelve years old. Blackpool was chosen, largely, I think, because Dad had been stationed there during the war, and had told us about the spectacular tower and the three piers. By that time my residual vision was very poor indeed, which probably accounts for an impression of grey mistiness. I did remember the donkeys, though, and the evocative sound of the gulls, and the waves, and the rather sinister laughing man at the pleasure beach.

Since the weekend that was arranged coincided with Bonfire Night, it was hoped that I could be filmed pressing the plunger which would start what promised to be a spectacular firework display, as well as viewing the lights and visiting the pleasure beach.

Although I waited with almost child-like impatience for Friday to arrive, I experienced once again that feeling, almost of guilt, that I had done absolutely nothing to deserve all these wonderfully generous things that were being done for me, and my anticipated pleasure was momentarily tinged with gloom. Having packed the cases, with warm clothes, and installed Grandad, yet again, to look after the dogs for the weekend, the gloomy feeling began to melt away, and by the time we reached the end of the busy motorway and saw signs for Fleetwood, where we were to stay, it had disappeared completely.

I thought Mary had been joking when she told me that Ian and I had been given the executive suite. When she appeared, to see if we were settling in, I was still sitting, somewhat bemused, trying to take in my surroundings. The enormously high padded bedhead looked to me, at first, like an arched church window, although once I had touched it I couldn't imagine how it had ever appeared so. That is the way it so often happens. I sit for a long time in a strange place, unable to make head or tail of the most everyday things; then, once I have touched them or the place becomes familiar, they are so obviously what they are that I feel rather embarrassed about not having known from the start. I certainly had no difficulty in identifying the beautiful fresh flowers and, in the fruit bowl, the rosiest, shiniest apples I have ever seen. I do hope the giant gift-wrapped box of chocolates really was for me. I have kept the rather special box as a souvenir, but the chocolates aren't in it any more, I'm afraid. Having met David, the director, and Anne, the assistant producer – a talented lady of many parts, as we were to discover next day – we all dined together, and went our various ways to bed. Mary and I sat for a long time, discussing the next day's crowded schedule.

I hardly slept, my mind was so full of all the exciting things we had talked of, and, just as I had nodded off, the clanking of the first early-morning tram startled me into complete wakefulness. Although it was an unfamiliar sound, it seemed normal and homely, conjuring up a picture of families breakfasting by bright coal fires, and reliable father-figures going off to work wearing sturdy shoes or boots and flat caps. It felt safe, like my childhood home.

After breakfast, we stepped out into the bitter coldness of the November day. And what a day! Somehow it embodied circumstances and episodes that strangely called to mind certain facets of my own life and circumstances.

The film crew, four men, were a lively bunch, full of good humour and anecdotes. Gren, the cameraman, was particularly good with the boys. I found the whole business of being involved in making a film, and all it entails, fascinating. All the individuals involved had their own special roles, and yet one could see each part dove-tailing into a whole. The efficiency and concentration with which they worked, the jargon of their trade, and their sensitive handling of the public – there were plenty of them around, at every stage – delighted me.

After a walk along the prom, closely pursued, of course, by Gren and his camera, we admired the multifarious items on offer in a rock shop – rock dummies, rock teeth and rock fruit abounded in profusion, much to Ben's delight. Since we were being filmed admiring and choosing them, the different items had to be unwrapped, and then of course somebody had to eat them up.

The stall with 'Kiss-Me-Quick' hats was literally an eye-opener. Ben tried on one after another, lost in a world of his own. That gave me quite a funny feeling watching my own young son having such a good time trying on the funny hats, all shapes and sizes. I felt that I had captured, there on that wind-blown sea-front, a small part of his childhood that I might easily have missed.

On to the oyster bar, where we held up business for some considerable time. Always, of course, the relentless camera was at our heels, and the little microphones Ian and I had clipped inside our coat collars were listening in to every chance remark we might make, including, I am quite sure, some snatches of conversation meant only for the family's ears. I had never seen oysters, and was surprised that they had such rough shells. I had expected that they would be round and smooth, like the pearls themselves, I suppose. Mary, who stood quietly by, obviously overheard me commenting on this and, in a thrice, there we were, surrounded by the crew, who were taking shots from all angles, while I imparted this piece of information four or five times, into the little eavesdropper on my collar.

I actually tasted an oyster, but thought it a disgusting thing. The stall and its owner were a wonderful sight to behold. I love the striped aprons butchers and fish-mongers wear. They have a really distinctive look, like drawing a line under certain words. Something particularly colourful caught my eye. It was a huge crab, and, once again I simply had to touch it, although I could see its bright shell and its shape well enough.

After lunch, we walked along the North Pier, where Russ Abbot, the well-known comedian, was to meet us. One of those seaside cardboard cut-outs of a fat lady had been set up on the pier; he was looking out through the hole where her face should be, as we came towards him, and he started talking as 'Jimmy', one of his characters, with a Scottish accent. For some unaccountable reason, this quite frightened me, and I was relieved when he stepped out and greeted us in his own voice. Not for the first time that day, a considerable crowd had gathered around us, attracted, of course, by the cameras. Ian did a wonderful public relations job, patiently answering their questions. We chatted to Russ Abbot for quite a long time. He joked, and made the boys laugh.

The public relations people at Blackpool and the BBC staff had made a most impressive job of organizing the day between them, so that one event flowed smoothly into another. Anne, the assistant producer, had a remarkable way of seeming to spirit cups of coffee and hot chocolate out of thin air, in response to our frequent requests. I am sure that her alacrity in so doing averted an attack of hypothermia in more than one of our number.

As dusk began to fall, we waited outside the tram garage, where we were to board the open-topped tram, for the ride along the famous Golden Mile. I actually began to feel nervous, with butterflies in my stomach. I longed to see the lights, about which I had heard so much. But what if I couldn't see them properly? I would feel terrible after all the trouble that had been taken on my behalf. I took some deep breaths, knowing that I can always make things out much more easily when I'm relaxed. It was exciting, sitting so high up on the tram, looking down on the world. The people on the pavement below looked like matchstick men, their legs being the part of their anatomy that I could most easily identify. As the tram drew out on to the front, I felt the cold sea-breeze on my cheeks, and I was glad that the inimitable Anne had thought to organize rugs and hot-water bottles for us. Suddenly, I wanted to stand up, and shout to everyone 'I've come to see the lights. I've really come to see them.' I didn't shout, thank goodness, but I did stand up, and look across to where the dark sea was, and felt a sort of affinity with it, as it rolled out towards the darkness of the unknown world beyond and back again towards the glitter and the brightness and noise. I knew all about that unremitting pull, tugging you first this way and then back again, not knowing quite which way to go, because you're not quite sure where you really belong.

Ian tugged my sleeve, and told me that our journey into the land of lights had begun. For the next hour, I hardly knew which way to look. Above, ahead, to the right and to the left, were lights, lights, lights. There we were, high up amid a fantastic, dazzling world of lights, which, bit by bit, came to mean something. At the side I picked out, quite quickly and easily, some that had a fairly simple, banner-like appearance. I found them pleasing, because it was possible for me to take in the idea of them without any effort. There were eye-catching lanterns, again easy to recognize, and, less easy, but beautiful, once I had sorted them out with Ian's help, colourful peacocks, which hung down the centre of the road. Strings and strings of lights, looped and threaded like never-ending strings of beads, reminding me again of the beaded handbags we carried to dances, years ago. There were intricate displays depicting well-known nursery rhymes and children's stories. They were almost lifelike, in a fantastic kind of way. There was Mickey Mouse, with his lovely big curved ears sticking up at a saucy angle. I recognized him easily. As a child, I used to have a Mickey Mouse comic on Sundays – I remember being able to see the pictures quite clearly, and the frustration at not being able to read for myself the stories that accompanied them. Now here were characters that meant nothing to me. Because, by the time I was able to see pictures again, our boys had outgrown them, such characters as Postman Pat and Yogi Bear, are only names to me.

There was so much to take in. Look here, look there. This way, that way. One fantastic sight followed another, and still more twinkled and shone ahead. There was an enchanting gingerbread house, made of sweets and biscuits. That was very pretty indeed. My head began to spin and, although my eyes went on looking, my brain suddenly refused to take in any more. However much I wanted to go on enjoying all these wonderful sights, my brain had had enough, and refused, for the time being, to interpret one more thing. All the same, it seemed the ride on the tram was over too soon. There was no doubt the illuminations had lived up to all my expectations. If I had seen half as much, my eyes would have had a feast-day.

Next a meal, then off we all went to the North Pier again. For many years, I had not been particularly thrilled by fireworks, although I can remember being able to see the brighter and larger ones. When the boys were small, we had some really good bonfire parties, and invited friends to share them with us. In recent years, though, I had usually stayed at home, on the pretext of looking after the dogs, while Ian and the boys went off to some locally organized event. My perception of light had deteriorated so much, during the last few years, that I could hardly see even the largest fireworks, and I hated their spluttering and banging.

The sky, that night in Blackpool, was very dark. The lighted tower pointed heavenwards like a jewelled finger. Suddenly the banging and spluttering reverberated in the chilly air, echoing the booming out across the sea. Oh yes, I jumped all right. As I looked across to where the noise had begun, I saw that the dark sky was now ablaze with twinkling, spinning, sparkling lights. Lights like waterfalls cascaded and tumbled in the air. Others seemed to burst and fall like showers of soft petals, floating down to the dark water. Great chrysanthemums of light filled the black space of the sky, falling eventually, as Ian remarked, like dandelion clocks, soft as thistledown. I was so mesmerized by the whole incredible spectacle that I quite forgot about the great explosions of noise, still echoing everywhere. As one magical display followed another, I was lost for words to describe the wonder of it all. And then, once again, quite suddenly, that was it: I couldn't take in any more. I had had enough. It had been a wonderful sight, a fantastic experience for me, but all at once it simply didn't register any more.

To round off our exciting, crazy, experience-packed day, we went to the famous pleasure beach. There was

the memorable sound of the laughing man, a life-sized
effigy, rocking and roaring with crazy laughter – I still
found it weird and strangely unpleasant. Everything
else, though, was light and bright, and just made for fun.
I watched children with sticks in their hands, topped
with enormous, wobbling, sugary-pink clouds of candy-
floss. Instead of just standing waiting, as I have quite
happily done for years, I stood watching. I watched the
faces, lit up by the brightness of the stalls. Just watching
others taking part, made me feel a part of it all. When,
however, at one of the stalls, I could see really clearly
rows of what looked like red, blue and yellow bottles,
which turned out to be skittles, I couldn't wait to have a
go. I actually lost count of the number of times I hurled
the little ball at the bright skittles, and it gave me the most
enormous amount of childish pleasure when I saw them
topple and go clattering down. When the stall-holder
announced that I had won a prize, and placed a toy koala
bear in my arms, I could barely contain my joy. I had
certainly never won a prize for anything like that before.
Trevor, for I named him after the friendly man at the
skittle stall, sits in state in our sitting-room. Later, at
Mary's invitation, he accompanied me to Pebble Mill,
where everyone respectfully referred to him as Trevor. I
do hope the man with the skittles saw him.

On Sunday morning, the plan was to meet again at the
North Pier for a ride in one of the old-fashioned horse-
drawn carriages. I had looked forward, too, to a trip up
the tower, to find out how much I could see from the
observation platform. But at ten o'clock that Sunday
morning thick, grey fog had wrapped itself around the
tower, the piers and the promenade, and hung there like
a great, drab, dank curtain. The film crew hung around
for an hour or so, and then decided that, even if the fog
should lift, which seemed highly unlikely, the light

would not be right for what they had been hoping to do. I was quite sad to see them go. After only twenty-four hours, I felt as though I had known them for years.

Mary and I had used the time to do some recording with the sound engineer. We sat there on the pier trying not to be conspicuous, if that's possible with a great furry microphone held in front of your face. I felt snug, in my warm boots and scarf and gloves, but shivered as the cries of seagulls came in a plaintive wail through the fog-laden air.

'Isn't it dingy and depressing?' I remarked. I could hardly believe that last night, from almost that spot, the sky had been a riot of light, and colour, and movement as far as one could see. Now, just murky, clinging, grey fog. Mary said it made her think of Cinderella.

'Yes, Cinderella.' I picked up her train of thought. 'That's exactly what it's like. Cinderella would look dingy and drab, in the daytime. Almost commonplace, I suppose, although I'm sure she'd have a warm heart. Then, all at once, there'd be such a transformation, right before your eyes. You'd blink, and when you opened your eyes again, there she'd stand in her glittering, glamorous ball-gown, ready for fun and laughter, and maybe even a little romance.'

It really was rather like that. On first seeing the tower, the previous day, I think I had been a little shocked by its stark appearance, surprised that I could see the sky through what looked like girders on a building site. I think I had expected it to be something like the spire of a church, probably made in stone. As I'd looked up at it, I had an uncanny feeling that it was leaning down towards me, and that, if I had stood on tiptoe, I could have reached up and touched it. At night, though, when it stood up, tall and softly illuminated, rising from a great riotous flood of dancing lights, it had looked almost regal, and I'd found myself looking back at it, over my shoulder, several times.

Towards lunchtime the sun suddenly broke brilliantly through the fog, but it was too late by then to go sightseeing from the top of the tower. We did have our ride, though. By now the sky was a beautiful shade of blue and, as I looked out across the beach to the sea, I was soothed by the gentle rocking motion of our open carriage. When we alighted, I was moved almost to tears, once again, by the great dark, shiny animal, with his enormous hoofs and his gracefully arched neck. He stood there so patiently between the shafts. That was a beautiful way to end a memorable and truly exciting weekend.

There had been a sort of symbolic significance about more than one thing, during that weekend. There we had stood, the dark sky giving no hint that it would be different in any way from any other winter's night. Then, suddenly, at the touch of a switch, with an explosion that left you wondering what had happened, the darkness was shattered, and its place taken by one great glittering display after another. But, between each visual feast, there was something poignant, like an echo, about the darkness that enveloped us once more, whose duration we had no way of measuring, before the next fiery spectacle banished the darkness.

Wasn't that, I reflected, much as my own life had been, since the day the dressings had been removed and, rather like an explosion, the half-forgotten dimension of sight had burst upon my brain? One fresh sight after another, after another. Some flamboyant, exotic, and even full of majesty and grandeur, others lovely because of their utter simplicity and ordinariness. Then the dreadful, dreary darkness, which from time to time had

descended, unwelcome, unsought, and little understood. And again, just when it seemed that that was it,
the show was over and the light would never return, like
the unexpected creations I had seen in the sky, a child's
smile at a bus stop, one of the dogs looking up with
trusting eyes, lights across the valley, or frost on a
cobweb, would set the whole world on fire, and glowing
with light again.

Epilogue

Another Christmas has come and gone, the second since my eyes reopened upon a world of movement, and colour, and bright beauty, still half-seen, half-understood.

The many wonderful experiences of the intervening year have in no way dulled the wonder of it all. Now, however, for most of the time, I feel that I have stepped off the whirling top on which my feet could never find a steady foothold. For quite a lot of the time, now, I know that I am me, and who that 'me' really is. Gradually I am coming to terms with the odd place where I have come to perch, between the worlds of seeing and not seeing. It is beginning not to matter that I do not see as others see, that, my fingers scanning the pages of a book in Braille and my working guide dog at my feet, I can look across a room and remark upon something that is completely visual. At last, after all this time, when someone says to me 'I don't know how much you can see', I can answer with complete honesty, and no longer embarrassed by it, 'Neither do I, but it doesn't worry me any more.' And, as I become more confident and relaxed in my still comparatively new situation, I find others around me relaxing, too.

Perhaps this year, even more than last, the things I saw will remain the most vivid memories of the season of goodwill. I could not take my eyes off the colourful decorations at St Andrew's School. I traced and retraced, time and time again, the shapes of paper garlands, stars and glittering streamers. Because I cannot see them well enough to spot their true identity, the tiny figures dressed as Joseph and Mary, angels, shepherds and kings, became almost the real thing for me. I peeped through the glass door of the school hall, again and again, to wonder at the brightly lit tree.

Of all the beautiful things that I have seen during the past year, there are few that bring a lump into my throat as does the simple, elegant shape of a Christmas tree, decked out in its brilliant festive finery. As I stood, with dozens of others, by the tree in the market place on Christmas Eve, I looked at the soft light from the coloured bulbs and was unaccountably moved, and glad that those around me were singing too lustily and enthusiastically to notice that half the time I couldn't join in with the singing, for being half choked by emotion. The most beautiful of all was the green and gold giant that stood, a graceful and glorious offering to God, at the front of our beautifully decorated church. The gentle light of dozens of flickering candles made a most fittingly lovely backdrop for the unfolding story of the Saviour's birth, as told in the Christmas readings and carols. And there, among the candlelight and music, I was moved to give silent thanks for the simple beauty of it all.

Ian and Ben decorated our sitting-room and tree about a week before Christmas. The living-room and hall looked bare in comparison. I knew that Ian would be very busy during the next few nights, and saw no reason why I shouldn't get on with it, with the help of Adam's height to fasten things to the ceiling. However, the decorations that were left in the box looked decidedly tired, and more than ready to be pensioned off, I decided. During our shopping trip, Victor and I went into one of the self-service stores in Belper. As usual, I asked another customer if she would find an assistant to help me. When she arrived, Victor and I followed her to the stand where the Christmas decorations were displayed – all neatly packed, of course, in plastic bags. My helper was very patient, and found several packets containing the kind of thing she thought I would like.

Then, to my surprise, she said, 'There are pictures on the packets of what they look like. See if you can see them.' She held them up in front of me. 'I'll have to hold them so that the light is right for me,' I explained. Without another word, the packets were handed to me, and, after twisting them round to catch the right light, I could see the illustrations quite well, and had a good idea of what I was buying. For me, this was a tremendous breakthrough, a small thing, maybe, in usual circumstances, but it was as though someone had taken a jug containing something called confidence and topped me up with it, giving my spluttering engine a new lease of life. That lady may probably never know just what she did for me that day. Adam and I decided where to hang the new decorations, and when Ian came home he was astonished by the transformation that had occurred during his absence.

The Post Office was not busy when I called one grey afternoon in December, so I asked if I could have a look at some Christmas wrapping paper. Within moments the counter was covered with such a profusion of bright colour that the grey sky was quite forgotten while, for the next twenty minutes or so, I turned over sheet after sheet, describing, to the delight of the sub-postmaster and his wife, the cheerful designs, all staring out at me in shades of red, blue, green and silver. As I chose the pieces I liked best, we chatted about how the tables had turned. Just two years before, they had had to describe the designs to me. Now, here I was, spelling out seasonal messages, identifying futuristic reindeer, and more traditional bells and trees, and even getting most of the colours right. I think Angela and Brian enjoyed the experience almost as much as I did.

We had a lovely family Christmas, with my parents and Ian's father to share it with us. During the days that followed, we visited and were visited by friends. What more could anyone ask? And yet there was one more treat to come. TV-am invited me to appear on the programme on the Wednesday following Christmas Day. This meant that Ian and I had to travel down to London on the Tuesday evening, and stay overnight. It was a nostalgic occasion – a poignant reminder of a year earlier, when everything had been so new and highly charged. Somehow, with a year's experience behind me, this time was even more special.

Before going to the hotel, we asked the driver who had brought us from Belper if we might look at the lights in the West End. I thought they were beautiful, but sophisticated and rather regal, rather than Christmassy and colourful like the ones at home. Suddenly, though, I was aware of the beautiful lines of a floodlit church, and was amazed that I was able to identify it correctly as St Martin-in-the-Fields. My visual memory is usually poor.

Watching *Mary Poppins* on television, on Christmas Eve, the close-up shots of St Paul's Cathedral had given me special delight. Ever since the grace and symmetry of its great dome against the night sky had made such an unexpected impact upon my brain, just one year before, I had thought about it often. When I think about the hard, unresponding feel of stone beneath my fingertips, it is almost unbelievable that, with human hands and crude tools, a thing of such indescribable and lasting beauty could have been created. 'Do you think we could have a quick look at St Paul's?' I ventured. A few moments later there it was, proud and spendid, a hiding place and

resting place for the secrets of the souls of men and
women who have chosen to leave them there.

Before returning home, after our early-morning visit to
the television studios, we went back to St Paul's and sat
in the nave for a long time, just looking and looking. The
way I felt then is too special, and too deep-down inside,
to describe in mere words. My emotions belonged to the
world of music, pure music, without words. I have no
idea how many steps we climbed, up to the top of the
dome, but the climb was as breathtaking as the view out
across the rooftops of the city, once we had arrived, legs
aching and too much Christmas fare telling its own tale,
out on the parapet. I was having a wonderful seeing day,
with not a trace of the obtrusive orange glare to mar my
view. Far below, what looked like a dull grey ribbon was,
Ian explained, the river. I couldn't understand why there
were so many enormously tall, thin chimneys, standing
at more or less equal distances from each other. These, it
turned out, were the high blocks of flats at the Barbican.
Nearby, far, far down, two bright spots, like large,
shining beads, on a triangle of green turned out to be two
street-lamps on a triangular lawn. Apart from these
specific things, it looked as though someone had taken
dozens and dozens of pieces of paper, all rectangular,
and mostly in shades of grey, some large and others
small, and had just scattered them in no particular order
as far as my eyes could see. These, I learned, were dozens
and dozens of rooftops of the houses and offices and
business premises of the City of London.

Imperfect though my view may have been from my
perch there, so high up on that glorious historic place, I
was thrilled to the very depths of my being. What I saw
was first-hand. I was seeing it. Chimneys or high-rise
flats; a grey ribbon or a river; a pack of grey cards,
haphazardly abandoned to fall wherever they would, or

the rooftops of the capital whose heartbeat I could feel through the ancient grey stonework against which my own heart was beating? It matters not. I was more than happy as I looked out through the narrow stone slit, and saw it all in my way. I am coming to think, more and more, that the important thing is not how much we see of things, but how much we can see in them. I am talking about the luxury of seeing. I believe that, even in my imperfect way, I have been privileged to drink to the depths of beauty's cup.

From the moment that the first dressings were removed, I have lived in a sort of perpetual Cinderella land, dressed one moment in rags and the next in glittering riches. When my eyes are bad, and my vision is marred by the orange glow, I am discouraged, and wonder why I didn't leave things alone, the way I had understood them for so long. All that changes in an instant as the curtain, almost without warning, is drawn aside, and I catch sight through my window of the river sparkling in the sun-light, or see the long, pearly reflections of street lights across the water. Then I gaze and gaze, and hope the midnight hour will not strike until my eyes have had enough of looking. The dark 'No-Man's-Land' days are not easy to cope with, and seem as though they will never end, dark among the cobwebs and the dust. Then, unexpectedly, the pumpkin becomes a glittering coach, the dingy dust is left behind, forgotten, and all is fun and laughter there among the gaiety and glitter of the ball.

My story has attracted much publicity – perhaps more than it should have, or than was wise. I do not know. My family, I am sure, have been little affected by it all: to them I am, as I should be, just Mum. Occasionally, when I have been off to the television studios in Birmingham and arrived home before the boys have come home from school, they have dismissed it completely from their minds, wanting to talk about far more important matters such as the football match they played in at lunchtime, or which team Derby County has drawn in the Cup match. Maybe one or two of my friends found it all a little difficult to cope with at the start, fearing that the publicity would change me, and go to my head. I don't suppose it has been easy for those who know where all the warts are, to cope with the magazine articles that always portray a perpetually smiling woman, who never yells at the dogs when she has tripped over one of them for the third time, never nags at her kids for going upstairs in muddy shoes or leaving wet towels on the bathroom floor. Not that I have tried to hide those truths, but the magazines don't seem to find them very interesting.

And my faith? It is still simple, and still strong. I do not pretend to understand the being whom I call God. I don't try to give reasons for disasters and cruelty and wars, because I do not understand them at all. I pray daily for hostages, abused children, and starving people, in the firm belief that prayers are heard, but without any understanding of why, sometimes, they appear to go unanswered. I believe that God answers prayers in his time, and in his way. Simplistic maybe, even trite, but that is what I believe, and I quarrel with no one's right to believe otherwise.

However imperfectly I may understand these immeasurably deep mysteries, there is one thing that I know for certain. What happened to me did not happen because I had either earned or deserved it. If that were the way blessings worked, I would probably be grovelling somewhere near the first rung of the ladder. I bow my head with genuine humility, perhaps even a little shame, when I hear for instance, of people with no limbs having the courage to go out in front of vast crowds to take part in competitive sports, or of others who, knowing themselves to be dying of dreadful terminal illnesses, instead of succumbing to understandable self-pity, use their remaining energies in the service of others. I am not a brave person. I will not even cross a field if I know there are cows or even sheep in it. I shall never climb a mountain, and would not dare to make a parachute jump. I believe myself to be very ordinary, just like most other people that I meet along life's way. Like them, I have known darkest sorrow, and walked along the darkest path in the deep valley – the path that is hardly touched by the sun's bright rays. And like them, I have sailed along on fast-moving clouds of ecstasy and joy, in a place where there is all light and no shadows.

What of my aspirations for the future? They are simple, probably even a little commonplace, and certainly not in the least adventurous. I hope that, when I give talks to groups and societies, clubs and schools, on the work of Guide Dogs for the Blind Association, I shall continue, in my small way, to open the eyes of those of my audience who do not already understand that disabled people are simply people like themselves. That, like them, they have hopes and aspirations. They may be courageous, bitter, humorous or sad – and different things at different times, because that is the way people are. Unfortunately, barriers do still exist, but I believe they exist because of embarrassment and lack of understanding, hardly ever through intentional unkindness. I suppose that, after my family, teaching is still my greatest love. I dared to hope once, when I was young and inexperienced, that someone would have enough faith to allow me to prove myself, and use whatever gift I might possess. They did, and I am grateful to them. Now, in the middle years of my life, mellowed by experience and a maturer understanding, I dare to hope again that a door will open somewhere, some day. Above all, though, I hope that, when I come to the end of my life, I shall be able to look back, and know that I have done at least one thing really well.

I am sometimes asked how I feel about the years that I spent in the darkness, or the shadows, or whatever blindness is. I am asked, too, if I am bitter that the light was not let in before. The answer is an unqualified and honest 'no'. The shadows were not so bad as you might imagine them to be. If the shadows, or darkness, had not existed, I would never have known the indescribable joy of seeing those three pairs of soft, dark eyes looking at me, in almost mystified unbelief, from the foot of my hospital bed. I would not have had the rare privilege of seeing, in adult life, Christmas trees, an upside-down world in the water, a cobweb with frost glistening upon it, hot-air balloons, a blackbird singing on a tree stump, and dozens of other wonderful things, through the ever-hungry, ever-awakening eyes of a child.